# *Mediterranean Diet*

## FOR DUMMIES®

A Wiley Brand

## *Pocket Edition*

by Meri Raffetto, RD, LDN and
Wendy Jo Peterson, MS, RD

D1205851

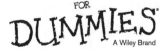

FOR DUMMIES®

A Wiley Brand

# Mediterranean Diet For Dummies® Pocket Edition

Published by
**John Wiley & Sons, Inc.**
111 River St.
Hoboken, NJ 07030-5774
www.wiley.com

Copyright © 2013 by John Wiley & Sons, Inc., Hoboken, New Jersey

Published simultaneously in Canada

For general information on our other products and services, please contact our Customer Care Department within the U.S. at 877-762-2974, outside the U.S. at 317-572-3993, or fax 317-572-4002.

For technical support, please visit www.wiley.com/techsupport.

Wiley publishes in a variety of print and electronic formats and by print-on-demand. Some material included with standard print versions of this book may not be included in e-books or in print-on-demand. If this book refers to media such as a CD or DVD that is not included in the version you purchased, you may download this material at http://booksupport.wiley.com. For more information about Wiley products, visit www.wiley.com.

ISBN 978-1-118-74814-5 (pbk); ISBN 978-1-118-74805-3 (ebk); ISBN 978-1-118-74815-2 (ebk); ISBN 978-1-118-74820-6 (ebk)

Manufactured in the United States of America

10 9 8 7 6 5 4 3 2 1

# Table of Contents

. . . . . . . . . . . . . . . . . . . . . . . . . . . . . . .

## Chapter 7: Starting and Ending with Style: Appetizers and Desserts ......................113

## Chapter 8: Ten Tips for Getting More Plant-Based Foods in Your Diet ...........................129

# Introduction

•  •  •  •  •  •  •  •  •  •  •  •  •  •  •  •  •  •  •  •  •  •  •  •  •  •  •

*I*magine the Mediterranean Sea, where the water and the land are big parts of life. Picture people eating fresh foods and relaxing with friends and family. That image is the essence of the traditional Mediterranean diet. The Mediterranean diet is part of certain lifestyle habits, including diet, physical activity, stress management, and fun, used in various regions of the Mediterranean coast. Research has shown that people who live in these areas have less heart disease and better longevity. Throughout this book, you discover how these habits affect your health and well-being.

We know that changing habits isn't easy. The life strategies we discuss can be challenging because they all focus on one main trend — slowing down — that's at odds with many people's busy lifestyles. Our goal is to show you that implementing a Mediterranean diet and lifestyle can be simple and flavorful. You don't have to follow a strict dietary plan or omit any foods; the Mediterranean diet is more about adding than taking away. This book is here to help you make small changes so you can find more balance in your life.

## About This Book

In the following pages, you find information about the Mediterranean region, the balance of foods the people there eat, the health benefits of this style of eating, and recipes full of delicious flavor. You also find some general cooking and meal-planning tips.

You can use this book as a resource, and you don't have to read it from cover to cover. Instead, you can find a new recipe to try or head straight to the chapter that contains the type of information you need.

# Conventions Used in This Book

We recommend that you read all the way through each recipe before you start making it. That way, you can account for any necessary refrigeration time, marinating time, and so on and for any special tools that the recipe may require. Here are a few other guidelines to keep in mind about the recipes in this book:

- ✔ All measurements are provided in standard weights and volumes. For help with metric conversions, please visit www.dummies.com/go/metricmeasure.

- ✔ All butter is unsalted unless otherwise stated. Margarine isn't a suitable substitute for butter.

- ✔ All eggs are large.

- ✔ All milk is lowfat unless otherwise specified.

- ✔ All onions are yellow unless otherwise specified.

- ✔ All pepper is freshly ground black pepper unless otherwise specified.

- ✔ All salt is kosher.

- ✔ All dry ingredient measurements are level.

- ✔ All temperatures are Fahrenheit.

- ✔ All lemon and lime juice is freshly squeezed.

- ✔ All sugar is white granulated sugar unless otherwise noted.

- ✔ All flour is all-purpose white flour unless otherwise noted.

Finally, we include the following basic conventions throughout the rest of the book:

- ✔ We use *italic* when we define a word or phrase.

- ☉ We use this little tomato icon to highlight vegetarian recipes.

- ✔ When we recommend websites, we haven't added any extra spaces or punctuation in them (even if they break over two lines), so type exactly what you see in the text.

# Foolish Assumptions

When writing this book, we made the following few assumptions about you, our dear reader:

- ✔ You're looking for meal-planning tips that will help you succeed with your health and weight-loss goals.

- ✔ You have an understanding of cooking basics, such as how to use a knife without cutting your finger. If you need to brush up on your cooking skills, check out *Cooking Basics For Dummies*, 4th Edition, by Bryan Miller, Marie Rama, and Eve Adamson (Wiley) before you get rolling.

- ✔ You're looking for ways to get more vitamins, minerals, and antioxidants into your diet.

- ✔ You're genuinely willing to make changes and stick to them until they become habits.

# Icons Used in This Book

The icons in this book are like bookmarks, pointing out information that we think is especially important. Here are the icons we use and the kind of information they point out:

Even if you forget everything else in this book, remember the paragraphs marked with this icon. They help you stay on track with your health goals.

 This helpful icon marks important information that can save you time and energy.

 Watch out for this icon; it warns you about potential problems and common pitfalls of implementing a Mediterranean diet into your lifestyle.

## *Where to Go from Here*

Where to go from here depends on your immediate needs. Looking for a great new dessert to make tonight? Head to Chapter 7. Interested in finding out more about the health benefits of the Mediterranean diet? Sit back and read Chapter 2. Want to get some ideas for how to stock your kitchen as you prepare to change your approach to cooking and eating? Check out Chapter 4.

If you're not sure where you want to begin, peruse the table of contents, pick out the topics that mean the most to you, and start there. Wherever you begin, we hope you find the information and inspiration you need to start making positive changes for your health.

To find even more advice on how to transition to a Mediterranean lifestyle, check out the full-size version of *Mediterranean Diet Cookbook For Dummies* — simply head to your local book seller or go to www. dummies.com!

# Chapter 1

# Journeying to Club Med: What's This Diet All About?

. . . . . . . . . . . . . . . . . . . . . . . . . . . . . . . .

*In This Chapter*

▶ Exploring the origins of the Mediterranean diet

▶ Focusing on Mediterranean lifestyle habits

▶ Peeking at the Mediterranean food guide pyramid

. . . . . . . . . . . . . . . . . . . . . . . . . . . . . . . .

*W*hen you picture the Mediterranean diet, you may imagine the sea lapping up on a beach near a quaint village whose residents are lounging and eating fresh grapes and olives. That picture is a good start.

The Mediterranean diet is a way of life — one where you eat lots of fresh food and slow down. More technically, the Mediterranean diet is a modern set of guidelines inspired by traditional diet patterns of southern Italy, the Greek island of Crete, and other parts of Greece. The lifestyle was first researched in the 1960s, and in 2010, the United Nations Educational, Scientific and Cultural Organization (UNESCO) officially recognized this diet pattern to be part of the cultural heritage of Italy, Greece, Spain, and Morocco. A more rural lifestyle is a common thread among all these regions.

Research shows that following a traditional Mediterranean diet significantly reduces the risk of heart disease, cancer, heart attack, and stroke. For example, in 2013 the website of the *New England Journal of Medicine* published results of a study of 7,447 people at high risk of having cardiovascular problems. Some study participants followed a Mediterranean diet — increasing their intake of plant-based foods, seafood, and healthy fats and decreasing intake of processed meat, red meat, and commercial baked goods, for example — and supplemented with olive oil. Others followed a Mediterranean diet and supplemented with nuts. A control group was asked to follow a lowfat diet (but actually didn't change its dietary habits much at all). Study results indicated that eating the traditional Mediterranean diet substantially reduced the risk of heart attack, stroke, and heart disease–related death among this high-risk population.

The key word here is *traditional*. The Mediterranean region is changing, with faster-paced lifestyles and more modern conveniences. These changes bring with them an increased prevalence of the ills we're trying to avoid.

For the purposes of this book, when you think of a Mediterranean lifestyle and dietary patterns, the focus is on the traditional habits seen at least 50 years ago in the regions we note here. For instance, if you visited northern Italy on a recent trip, you may not have experienced any of the dietary patterns we promote in this book. So no, that huge portion of butter-laden pasta you had doesn't qualify for this diet.

Although diet is a big component of the health benefits experienced in the Mediterranean, all the lifestyle patterns combined, including physical activity and relaxation, may provide insight into the health benefits found in this region. This chapter serves as your jumping-off point into the Mediterranean diet and breaks down the Mediterranean dietary patterns and lifestyle choices that you can use as strategies for your own healthy lifestyle.

# Identifying the Flavors of the Mediterranean Coast

The Mediterranean Sea is actually part of the Atlantic Ocean; a total of 21 countries have a coastline on the Mediterranean. However, only a few truly epitomize the Mediterranean diet and lifestyle that we discuss in this book. Having a decent understanding of these countries and their cooking styles can help you have a better appreciation for this way of life.

The recipes in this book are inspired by Mediterranean cooking — specifically, the areas of southern Italy, Greece, Morocco, and Spain. Although you may see some of the same ingredients in many recipes, the flavors used in different countries or regions create entirely different dishes. For example, if you've eaten both Italian and Greek meatballs, you know that the two varieties sure don't taste the same. Table 1-1 lists some of the countries in the Mediterranean that are part of this lifestyle and the associated flavors and cooking styles commonly used in those areas.

| Table 1-1 | | Common Mediterranean Flavors by Region |
|---|---|---|
| **Region** | **Commonly Used Ingredients** | **Overall Cuisine Flavor** |
| Southern Italy | Anchovies, balsamic vinegar, basil, bay leaf, capers, garlic, mozzarella cheese, mushrooms, olive oil, oregano, parsley, peppers, pine nuts, prosciutto, rosemary, sage, thyme, tomatoes | Italian food is rich and savory, with strongly flavored ingredients. Look for tomato-based sauces and even an occasional kick of spicy heat. |
| Greece | Basil, cucumbers, dill, fennel, feta cheese, garlic, honey, lemon, mint, olive oil, oregano, yogurt | Greek cooking runs the gamut from tangy with citrus accents to savory. Ingredients such as feta cheese add a strong, bold flavor, while yogurt helps provide a creamy texture and soft flavor. |
| Morocco | Cinnamon, cumin, dried fruits, ginger, lemon, mint, paprika, parsley, pepper, saffron, turmeric | Moroccan cooking uses exotic flavors that encompass both sweet and savory, often in one dish. The food has strong flavors but isn't necessarily spicy. |
| Spain | Almonds, anchovies, cheeses (from goats, cows, and sheep), garlic, ham, honey, olive oil, onions, oregano, nuts, paprika, rosemary, saffron, thyme | Regardless of what part of Spain you're in, you can always count on garlic and olive oil setting the stage for a flavorful dish. Spanish dishes are often inspired by Arabic and Roman cuisine with emphasis on fresh seafood. You often find combinations of savory and sweet flavors, such as a seafood stew using sweet paprika. |

# Discovering Where the Food Comes From

Although you may be used to cruising to the grocery store and buying whatever you need, folks on the Mediterranean coast 50 years ago didn't roll that way. Instead, they depended on what was farmed and fished locally, making culinary specialties by using everything on hand. Those habits may be fading, but they're still the cornerstone of the Mediterranean diet, and you can still embrace them by incorporating fresh foods into your meals even if you don't live near the Mediterranean.

The following sections highlight where people in the Mediterranean get their food and why these strategies are so important.

## Focusing on farming

A moderate climate of wet winters and hot summers makes many of the areas along the Mediterranean ideal for agriculture. As a result, people living in the Mediterranean area can grow their own food in gardens and small farms, and many do so. This type of climate (similar to the climate of southern coastal California) also makes growing specialized foods like olives and fig trees easier, thus providing ingredients for some of the signature recipes from this region.

Many people in the Mediterranean also abundantly use fresh herbs, spices, onions, and garlic to provide big flavor to their cooking. Following is a partial list of common foods grown on the Mediterranean coast:

- ✔ **Legumes:** Chickpeas, lentils, peas
- ✔ **Fruits:** Figs, grapes, lemons, Mandarin oranges, olives, persimmons, pomegranates

✔ **Grains:** Barley, corn, rice, wheat

✔ **Herbs:** basil, dill, fennel, mint, oregano, parsley, rosemary, sage, thyme

✔ **Nuts:** Almonds, hazelnuts, pine nuts, walnuts

✔ **Vegetables:** Artichokes, asparagus, broccoli, broccoli rabe, cabbage, eggplant, garlic, green beans, onions, tomatoes

## *Eating seasonally*

As a side effect of eating what they grow locally, folks in the Mediterranean also eat seasonally; after all, you can't eat what you can't grow. Eating in-season food makes an impact for the following reasons:

✔ **Seasonal abundance makes you cook more creatively.** If you have an abundant amount of, say, green beans, you want to utilize them in any way possible. Finding different, tasty ways to prepare green beans as a side dish or as part of an entree requires more of a thought process, and more care goes into the food itself.

✔ **You eat an increased variety of produce throughout the year.** You may eat a lot of one food while it's in season, but when that season's over, you switch to other foods associated with the new time of year. In contrast, relying on produce available year-round at the grocery store means you can easily get stuck in a rut of eating the same standbys throughout the year.

More variety in produce means more variety of health-promoting nutrients that help you prevent disease. Although eating a few different types of fruits and vegetables throughout the year is better than nothing, getting a wide variety is the ultimate goal for good health.

We know that eating seasonally isn't feasible for many people in certain climates. But by actively seeking out locally grown foods at farmers' markets or in your grocery store, you can make choices that help you align more with this approach to cooking and eating.

## Fishing the Mediterranean Sea

People in the Mediterranean area rely on the nearby sea as a food source. Fish appear in many common traditional recipes, providing an abundance of healthy omega-3 fatty acids. You can add seafood to a few weekly meals and reap the same benefits. The least expensive seafood in the Mediterranean region includes sardines, anchovies, mackerel, squid, and octopus. Mid-priced fish and shellfish include tuna, trout, clams, and mussels. For a pricey, special-occasion meal, options include lobster and red mullet.

# Eating and Living the Mediterranean Way

The Mediterranean diet includes a specific balance of foods that's high in vitamins, minerals, and antioxidants and contains the perfect balance of fatty acids. Alas, you can't just eat your way to Mediterranean health. Living a healthy lifestyle means you have to look at all aspects of your life. Along with the food plan is a way of life that includes regular physical activity and time for rest, community, and fun; for the folks on the Mediterranean coast, this combination seems to have created that ever-elusive life balance.

To tie all the Mediterranean diet and lifestyle concepts together, Oldways Preservation and Exchange Trust (www.oldwayspt.org) came up with the Mediterranean Food Guide Pyramid based on the dietary traditions of Crete, other parts of Greece, and southern Italy around 1960, when chronic diseases such as heart disease and cancer were low. As you can see in Figure 1-1, the focus is on eating a diet rich in vegetables, fruits, whole grains, legumes, and sea-food; eating less meat; and choosing healthy fats such as olive oil. Note also the importance of fun activities, time shared with family and friends, and a passion for life. The following sections examine each aspect so that you can find it, too.

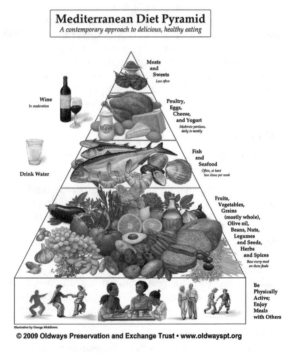

© 2009 Oldways Preservation and Exchange Trust • www.oldwayspt.org

**Figure 1-1:** The Mediterranean Food Guide Pyramid.

## *Focusing on healthy fats*

Although Mediterranean residents don't consume a lowfat diet, their dietary pattern is considered heart-healthy. How can that be? Not all fats are created equal. People in the Mediterranean consume more of the healthier types of fats (monounsaturated fats and polyunsaturated omega-3 fatty acids) and less of the omega-6 polyunsaturated fatty acids and saturated fats other cultures tend to overload on. Instead of focusing on total fat intake, these folks maintain a healthier ratio of these different groups of fats than you see in the United States; they consume about 35 percent of their total daily calories from fat, but less than 8 percent of their calories come from saturated fats. According to the National Health and Nutrition Examination Survey, the average intake of saturated fats in the United States is 11 percent of daily calories. You can find out more about the details of this fat ratio in Chapter 2.

To start rebalancing your fat ratio, limit your use of fats such as butter and lard in cooking and use more olive oils or avocadoes for spreads.

## *Using dairy in moderation*

You may think of the Mediterranean as a cheese-eater's heaven, but the truth is that the Mediterranean areas we focus on don't consume an abundance of cheese. Dairy is consumed on a daily basis in the Mediterranean diet, and cheese (along with yogurt) is a common source of calcium; however, moderation is the key (isn't it always?).

Incorporate two to three servings of dairy products daily. One serving may include an eight-ounce glass of milk, eight ounces of yogurt, or an ounce of cheese. Stick with the lowfat versions of milk and yogurt to help lower your saturated fat intake; because you're eating so little of it, you can go with regular cheese if you want.

## Eating primarily plant-based foods

One of the most important concepts of the Mediterranean diet pattern is consuming tons of plant foods such as fruits, veggies, legumes, and whole grains. People in the Mediterranean commonly eat five to ten servings of fruits and vegetables each day, which often means having two to three vegetable servings with each meal. Other daily staples include legumes such as beans, lentils, and peas, and whole grains such as bulgur wheat or barley.

Foods in these categories are naturally low in calories and high in nutrients, which makes weight- and health-management easy. Begin by finding ways to incorporate more unprocessed plant foods in your diet on a daily basis; Chapter 8 can help.

## Punching up the flavor with fresh herbs and spices

Fresh herbs and spices not only add tremendous flavor to food but also have many hidden health benefits, which we cover in Chapter 4. If you already use ample herbs and spices in your own cooking, you're on the right track. If not, this book can help you discover new flavors and simple ways to add more of these plants into your diet.

## Enjoying seafood weekly

Seafood is a weekly staple in the Mediterranean diet, and with good reason. Not only is it a local product (see the earlier section "Fishing the Mediterranean

Sea"), but also it's a great source of those coveted omega-3 fatty acids. If you live near a coast, you have a great opportunity to find fresh fish in your local stores and restaurants. If you're landlocked, don't discount lakes and rivers for fresh fish.

Check out www.montereybayaquarium.org/cr/ seafoodwatch.aspx for a list of recommended fish in your region. This guide is a great tool to help you choose local fish with low contaminants and also to protect against overfishing.

Don't like fish? You can get omega-3 fatty acids in other ways, such as with fish oil supplements or by eating lots of fresh herbs, walnuts, and flaxseeds.

## Limiting red meat

Red meat used to be a luxury item in rural parts of the Mediterranean, so folks there ate it less frequently. Even though it's now more accessible to the average Joe, the serving limits have stuck over the years.

Beef is served only once or twice a month in the Mediterranean rather than several times a week like in many U.S. kitchens. And when it does hit the table, it's usually as a small (two- to three-ounce) side dish rather than an eight-plus-ounce entree. This habit helps ensure a reasonable intake of saturated fats and omega-6 fatty acids. (See the earlier section "Focusing on healthy fats" for info on balancing fat intake.)

Don't panic at the idea of cutting your meat portion so drastically. You can easily replace some of that meat with lentils or beans to add plant-based protein to your meals, or add more vegetable servings to help fill the plate. Also keep in mind that Mediterranean beef recipes are so full of flavor that a small serving becomes more satisfying.

## *Having a nice glass of vino*

Wine lovers, rejoice! Drinking a glass of wine with dinner is certainly a common practice in the Mediterranean regions. Red wine has special nutrients that are shown to be heart-healthy; however, moderation is so important. Enjoying some red wine a couple times a week is certainly a good plan for heart health, although you want to check with your doctor to ensure it's okay for you. Check out Chapter 2 for specifics on the benefits of red wine.

## *Getting a good dose of daily activity*

Historically, the people in the rural Mediterranean got plenty of daily activity through work, getting where they needed to go on foot, and having fun. Although you may rely heavily on your car and think this lifestyle isn't realistic for you, you can still find ways to incorporate both aerobic exercise (which gets your heart rate up) and strength-training exercises regularly.

### Now that's a long weekend!

If you don't believe that slowing down can really do that much for your health, consider this study. Researchers from the University of Rochester found that from Friday night until Sunday, study participants, even those with high income or exciting work lives, were in better moods, showed greater enjoyment in life, and had fewer aches and pains. Having unscheduled time on the weekends provided individuals with opportunities to bond with others, explore interests, and relax. Hey, wait; those are some of the main tenets of the Mediterranean lifestyle! And if just a couple of days of downtime can make a difference, think about the effects of making this type of time a priority throughout the week.

Walking encompasses both aerobic and strength training and helps relieve stress. If you live close to markets or restaurants, challenge yourself to walk to them rather than drive, or simply focus on taking a walk each day to unwind.

## Taking time for the day's biggest meal

Even though the Mediterranean residents of days gone by were hard workers, often doing a significant amount of manual labor, they always made time for their largest meal of the day. Traditionally, this meal was lunch, where people sat down as a family and enjoyed a large meal full of vegetables, legumes, fruits, and seafood or meat. Taking time for meals and family was a priority; you didn't see people eating in five minutes at the countertop.

In many cultures, having this large relaxing meal at lunchtime is difficult because of work schedules. However, you can adapt this strategy into your life by focusing on supper. Prioritizing some time to unwind and relax from a busy work day provides other benefits for your family. According to a Columbia University survey, teenagers who eat with their families at least five days a week have better grades in school and are less prone to substance abuse.

 Although taking time for a large, relaxing meal sounds like one of those optional strategies you can skip, keep in mind that even small lifestyle choices can make a very big impact on overall health. Family dinners can help you clear your head from work and provide enjoyment through good food and conversation. If you're go, go, go all day at work, prioritizing family meal time can be priceless for your daily stress management.

# Fighting stress with daily rituals

Many principles of the Mediterranean lifestyle revolve around family, community, and fun. It's so easy to get caught up in a busy, hectic life and put these small experiences on the back burner because they don't appear to be that important. However, these little rituals throughout the day add up for a big impact on stress management. Stress impacts your health in so many ways, from increasing your risk of high blood pressure and heart disease to promoting weight gain, so managing it is key. Here are two examples of daily routines that illustrate how little experiences sprinkled throughout the day can provide more stress relief:

**1. Using Mediterranean lifestyle strategies**

✔ Wake up and have a light breakfast

✔ Workday begins (stress inducer)

✔ Lunch break with a light walk (stress reliever)

✔ End work day

✔ Home for sit-down dinner with family (stress reliever)

✔ Clean-up and evening tasks, such as kids' homework

✔ Reading or journaling (stress reliever)

✔ Bedtime (stress reliever)

In this example, the person has opportunities to let go of a little stress multiple times during the day. Now take a look at an example far too many people get trapped in:

**2. Using fast-paced lifestyle strategies**

✔ Wake up and skip breakfast (stress inducer)

✔ Workday begins (stress inducer)

✔ Lunch break, eating quickly in ten minutes at the desk (neutral — doesn't induce stress or reduce it)

✔ Work late (stress inducer)

✔ Rush through the drive-through to pick up a meal for family, eating in five minutes at the countertop (neutral)

✔ Clean-up and evening tasks, such as kids' homework

✔ Television (may be a stress inducer or reliever)

✔ Bedtime (stress reliever)

The first example has one big stress inducer (work) and four stress relievers sprinkled throughout the day. The second example has three to four stress inducers and only one or two stress relievers. That stress builds up in your body, setting you up for an increased risk of disease and possible weight gain. Taking the time for those small experiences during the day, such as a family dinner or a walk, make a big difference. And remember that the activities here are just examples. You can find stress relievers that work for you, such as knitting, yoga, tea time, painting, meditation, exercise, or conversation with a dear friend.

## *Enjoying time with friends and family*

Community spirit is a large part of the Mediterranean culture and is something that's disappearing in American culture. Getting together on a regular basis with friends and family is an important priority for providing a sense of strong community and fun. The fun and laughter that come with friendly get-togethers are vital for stress management. Without these little joyful experiences, stress can tip to an unhealthy balance.

To put this strategy into practice, invite some of your close family and friends over each week, perhaps for dinner. It can be as casual as you like. The important thing is to add this type of fun and enjoyment to your life more often.

## *Having a strong passion for life*

The Mediterranean coast is full of sunshine, good food, and beautiful surroundings, so the people who live there naturally tend to have a strong passion for life, family, friends, nature, and food. Choosing to have a strong passion and love of life is associated with more happiness and fulfillment and less stress.

What are you passionate about? Perhaps you love the arts, or maybe nature is your thing. Whatever your passions are, make sure to find a way to make them a part of your life.

# Chapter 2

# Savoring the Benefits of Eating Mediterranean

· · · · · · · · · · · · · · · · · · · · · · · · · · · · · · · · · · · ·

### *In This Chapter*

▶ Spotting powerful nutrients found in simple foods

▶ Toasting to the health benefits of red wine

▶ Highlighting heart health research

▶ Dealing with cancer and diabetes through diet

▶ Looking and feeling your best with anti-aging tips

· · · · · · · · · · · · · · · · · · · · · · · · · · · · · · · · · · · ·

*T*he Mediterranean diet has long been touted for providing health benefits, such as reducing coronary artery disease and decreasing the risk of some cancers. Including fresh vegetables and fruits, legumes, and healthy fats into your diet can help improve your health in many ways. And in addition to the health benefits, you're eating foods with full flavor. (Greek food and Italian food are rarely bland or boring.)

This chapter highlights why this diet is full of health benefits (focusing on heart disease, cancer, diabetes, and anti-aging) by looking at some of the main nutrients found in Mediterranean eating.

As you read this chapter, note that a healthy diet, exercise, and stress management can significantly reduce your risk of certain diseases, but nothing can bring a guarantee. Genetic components also play a role with chronic diseases. However, if you have family history of heart disease, diabetes, or cancer, incorporating these lifestyle and diet changes into your daily life can help you decrease those risks.

# Highlighting the Main Nutrients of the Mediterranean Diet

A plant-based diet such as the Mediterranean diet offers a plethora of nutrients that can help your body stay healthy. These plant foods are loaded with vitamins, minerals, antioxidants, phytochemicals, and healthy fats. The following sections highlight some of the key nutrients found in the foods associated with the Mediterranean coast.

## Fighting free radicals with antioxidants

*Antioxidants* are a key component of many plant foods that help slow down the process of oxidation (when your body's cells burn oxygen). This slowing decreases the amount of *free radicals,* or unstable molecules, that cause damage to your cells, tissues, and DNA. Antioxidants are a crucial part of your diet because you can't avoid oxidation altogether. Consider the many contaminants, such as car exhaust, sunlight, unhealthy foods, and air pollution, that you're exposed to during a typical day. These types of exposures can cause free radicals to gain speed in your body, damaging everything in their path and leaving you at greater risk of chronic conditions like heart disease and cancer.

Think about slicing an apple. Before you know it, the exposed flesh turns from white to brown. This browning occurs because of oxidation. But adding orange juice or lemon juice to the apple right after you slice it keeps it whiter longer because the antioxidant vitamin C in the juice protects the flesh.

Eating a diet high in antioxidants such as vitamin C, vitamin E, and beta-carotene means better protection for your body and overall health. The ATTICA study in the September 2005 issue of the *American Journal of Clinical Nutrition* measured the total antioxidant capacity of men and women in Greece. It found that the participants who followed a traditional Mediterranean diet had an 11 percent higher antioxidant capacity than those who didn't adhere to a traditional diet. The findings also showed that the participants who followed the traditional diet the most had 19 percent lower oxidized LDL (bad cholesterol) concentrations showing a benefit in reducing heart disease.

You don't have to look far or even cook that much to get antioxidants into your diet. You can find plenty of antioxidants in fruits and vegetables. If you're eating only one to three servings of fruits and vegetables per day, you need to increase your intake to take advantage of the produce's antioxidants. We challenge you to increase your intake of fresh fruits and vegetables to five to eight servings daily! The following list shows some common foods that are rich in certain antioxidants:

✔ **Vitamin C:** Asparagus, broccoli, cantaloupe, cauliflower, collard greens, grapefruit, green and red bell peppers, guava, kale, lemons, oranges, pineapple, spinach, strawberries, tangerines, tomatoes

✔ **Vitamin E:** Almonds, collard greens, mustard greens, peanuts, spinach, sunflower seeds, Swiss chard, turnip greens

✔ **Beta carotene:** Broccoli, cantaloupe, carrots, cilantro, collard greens, kale, romaine lettuce, spinach, turnip greens

## *Eating colorfully to get phytochemicals*

Besides vitamins and minerals, plants also contain phytochemicals. Don't be scared by the big word. *Phytochemicals* are simply healthy chemicals that offer your body healthful benefits. As we say repeatedly throughout this book, a plant-based diet high in fruits, vegetables, and legumes can provide you with an increased amount and variety of phytochemicals, helping to promote heart health and working to prevent certain cancers.

Research in this area is relatively new and is uncovering a whole side of previously unknown health benefits. To date, certain phytochemicals have been shown to work as antioxidants (see the previous section), contain anti-inflammatory properties, and promote heart health.

Phytochemicals provide the pigment to your fruits and vegetables, so you can literally know which class of phytochemicals you're consuming simply by noting the color you're eating. Table 2-1 shows a few specific health benefits found in each color.

# To supplement or not to supplement? That's still the question

Although you've likely heard the news that antioxidants found in foods promote good health, scientists are still researching whether taking supplements such as beta carotene, vitamin C, vitamin E, or other antioxidant blends can replace eating the real thing.

Research has provided a great deal of information about many individual nutrients and their impacts on health, but researchers still don't have the answers to many questions, such as how much of a supplement is enough and whether supplemented antioxidants have the same effect working on their own as the natural ones do working with accompanying nutrients. For instance, many fruits are high in vitamin C, so you may think that you can get the same vitamin C effects from taking a supplement if you don't eat a lot of fruit. However, the vitamin C in an orange may work with the phytochemicals in the orange to more significantly affect your health than the vitamin C supplement does by itself. Even supplements made from fruits and vegetables may not contain the other nutrients.

Another supplement concern is that taking high doses of antioxidants may actually cause the antioxidants to work as prooxidants that promote rather than neutralize oxidation. And in some cases, you actually want free radicals to attack harmful cells such as bacteria and cancer cells. High doses of antioxidant supplements may interfere with this natural process.

The bottom line is that eating whole foods is still your best bet to combat diseases and live your healthiest life. As we note throughout the book, folks in the Mediterranean eat scads of produce, and this type of food intake is one of the reasons you see more longevity in people who live in this region.

| Table 2-1 | Potential Health Benefits of Foods by Color | |
|-----------|---------------------------------------------|---|
| **Color** | **Health Benefits** | **Foods** |
| Blue/purple | A lower risk of some cancers; improved memory; and healthy aging | Blueberries, eggplants, plums, and purple grapes |
| Green | A lower risk of some cancers; healthy vision; and strong bones and teeth | Broccoli, green peppers, honeydew melon, kiwi, salad greens, and spinach |
| Red | A lower risk of heart disease and of some cancers, and improved memory function | Pink watermelon, red bell peppers, and strawberries |
| White | A lower risk of heart disease and of some cancers | Bananas, garlic, and onions |
| Yellow/orange | A lower risk of heart disease and of some cancers; healthy vision; and a stronger immune system | Carrots, oranges, yellow and orange bell peppers, and yellow watermelon |

## Vitamin D: Getting a little of the sunshine vitamin

Your body gets vitamin D, otherwise known as the sunshine vitamin, both from food sources and from exposure to sunlight. You want to make sure you get the appropriate amount of vitamin D; people in the Mediterranean may be healthier because they have strong levels of the vitamin.

The scientific community has been buzzing in the last ten years about the health benefits of vitamin D. Research shows this vitamin can help

✔ Protect against osteoporosis

✔ Reduce the risk of coronary artery disease

✔ Decrease the risk of certain cancers

✔ Lower the risk of infectious diseases such as the common flu

One theory suggests that the people of the Mediterranean coast are healthier because they're exposed to more sunlight — specifically, the ultraviolet B rays that are responsible for producing vitamin D — because they're outside more often walking, gardening, working, or enjoying family and friends.

To produce vitamin D, you want exposure to sunlight for 15 minutes each day with no sunscreen (sunscreen blocks up to 90 percent of vitamin D production). Of course, unprotected sun exposure increases the risk of skin cancer, so you have to weigh the good with the bad. Note that many people don't make enough vitamin D from the sun, including those who have darker skin tones, are overweight, are older, or live in northern climates.

In addition to the sun, you can get vitamin D from a few foods, such as fish, fortified cereals, and fortified milk. Food sources are limited, so you mostly need to depend on sun exposure to get the proper amounts.

Researchers agree that people's vitamin D levels need to increase, although the level of increase is still up for debate. In 2010, the Institute of Medicine released a report recommending the following daily intake of vitamin D:

✔ People ages 1 to 70 should take 600 IU (international units) a day.

✔ People over the age of 70 should take 800 IU (international units) a day.

 You can easily get your vitamin D levels checked with a simple blood test at your annual physical. Just let your primary care provider know if you have concerns about your level. Many people need to add a supplement to ensure they're getting the daily dose they need, but don't try to guess how much you need; taking too much vitamin D can have harmful consequences. Check out *Vitamin D For Dummies* by Alan L. Rubin, MD (Wiley) for more information.

## Choosing healthy fats

The Mediterranean diet is lower in omega-6 polyunsaturated fats (or *fatty acids*) and saturated fats than most people's diets are; it's also higher in healthy fats, such as monounsaturated fats and omega-3 polyunsaturated fats. (For reference, you find monounsaturated fats in foods such as olive oil, avocadoes, and certain nuts. Polyunsaturated fatty acids are in corn, safflower, soybean, sesame, and sunflower oils and seafood. Saturated fatty acids appear in animal-based foods such as meat, poultry, butter, and dairy products, as well as in coconut and palm oils.) The higher percentage of monounsaturated fats found in the Mediterranean diet is associated with

✔ A lower risk of heart disease

✔ Lower cholesterol levels

✔ Decreased inflammation in the body

✔ Better insulin function and blood sugar control

Omega-3 fatty acids are one of the big contributors to the health benefits of the Mediterranean diet, and many people don't get enough of them. Research shows that omega-3s help reduce inflammation, which is specifically important for those with inflammatory diseases such as arthritis, cardiovascular disease, or inflammatory bowel disease. These fats are also shown to be helpful for immune system function, behavioral issues such as attention deficit (hyperactivity) disorder, mood disorders such as depression, and prevention of Alzheimer's disease.

Omega-6 fatty acids occur abundantly in the diet through sources such as grains, nuts, and legumes as well as sunflower, safflower, sesame, and corn oils. Animal protein is also high in a specific omega-6 fatty acid called *arachidonic* acid. Omega-6 fats lower cholesterol, help keep the blood from clotting, and support skin health. Both omega-3 and omega-6 fats are considered *essential,* which means your body doesn't make them and needs to get them from your diet.

The big trouble begins when omega-3s aren't balanced appropriately with omega-6s. Although your omega-6 intake should be higher than your omega-3 intake, a diet too high in omega-6 fatty acids and too low in omega-3 fatty acids can promote conditions of chronic inflammation, including atherosclerosis, arthritis, and inflammatory bowel disease. Preliminary research also shows a possible connection to obesity, depression, dyslexia, and hyperactivity. This out-of-balance fat intake is very common in the American diet (with a ratio of 20 omega-6s to 1 omega-3) and less common in a Mediterranean style diet. Experts say the ratio to shoot for is about 4 parts omega-6 and 1 part omega-3.

Rebalance your diet by incorporating more sources of omega-3s, such as fresh herbs, canola oil, walnuts, flaxseeds, and cold-water fish (such as salmon, herring, and sturgeon), into your meals. You can also find products (such as eggs) fortified with omega 3s. Limit other sources of animal proteins (such as beef, poultry, unfortified eggs, and pork) by reducing your portion sizes to two to three ounces.

You can also repair the balance by replacing your cooking oils with olive oil, which is high in a third fat called omega-9 fatty acids. Your body can make omega-9s on its own, but adding more of them to your diet can help you lower your omega-6 intake.

## *Boosting your fiber intake*

"Eat more fiber." You've probably seen this message in advertisements and the media. You can get all the fiber you need by eating the Mediterranean way, focusing on fruits, vegetables, whole grains, and legumes.

Fiber is what you may call the "roughage" found in plants. Your body doesn't digest fiber like it does nutrients; fiber goes through your gastrointestinal tract intact. This process has a bigger impact on health than you may think. Here's what fiber can do for you:

- ✔ Help maintain a healthy gastrointestinal tract by decreasing constipation and reducing your risk of *diverticulosis,* or small pouches that form in your colon.

- ✔ Lower total cholesterol and bad cholesterol levels, helping to keep your heart healthy. This is the role played by the soluble fiber found in foods such as oat bran, beans, and flaxseeds.

- ✔ Slow the absorption of sugars you consume from carbohydrate foods, which helps keep blood sugar stable. This function is important for those who have insulin resistance diseases, such as diabetes or PCOS, and helps people manage their weight more effectively.

> ✔ Act as a natural appetite suppressant, helping you to feel full and satisfied after a meal. No need to buy those diet pills that are supposed to suppress your appetite. Save your money and try eating more fresh produce, beans, and whole grains with every meal.

# Understanding the Importance of Wine

Drinking more red wine, like many people in the Mediterranean coast do, may be one reason you're excited about switching to a Mediterranean diet. Red wine has certain properties that research has shown are beneficial for heart health. If you drink alcohol in moderation, add a little red wine in place of other alcoholic beverages. (If you're not a fan of red wine, drinking grape juice made from Concord grapes and eating purple grapes also provide similar heart-health benefits.)

The cardio protection red wine provides is attributed to the antioxidants from *flavonoids* found in the skin of the grapes. The flavonoids reduce your risk of heart disease by lowering bad cholesterol, increasing good cholesterol, and reducing blood clotting. A specific flavonoid called *resveratrol* may have additional benefits, including inhibiting tumor development in certain cancers, but that research is still in early stages.

Although red wine can indeed be part of a healthy lifestyle, a fine line determines what amount is considered healthy. The recommended daily intake is one 4-ounce glass for women and one to two 4-ounce glasses for men. Excessive drinking can become unhealthy and is linked to high blood pressure, cardiovascular conditions, and extra calories.

## Getting the facts about sulfites in wine

*Sulfites* are used as preservatives in many food products and also occur naturally in foods. Many people have sensitivities and allergies to sulfites, causing asthma-like symptoms, hives, and swelling. The headache that commonly results from drinking wine may be due to sulfite sensitivity, but it's more likely a question of overindulgence, dehydration, or lack of food in your stomach while drinking. If your headaches aren't consistent when you drink wine, you can't blame the sulfites (sorry). The best way to determine whether you have an allergy is to get yourself tested by an allergist, especially if you already suffer from asthma.

Sadly, you won't have much luck finding a sulfite-free wine; grape skins themselves are high in sulfites, and more are added in winemaking to give your wine a long shelf life. Without added sulfites, you get vinegar in a few months. Despite popular belief, European wines don't have fewer sulfites; in some cases, they have more!

You also need to be in good health to enjoy this perk of the Mediterranean diet. If you have high blood pressure, high triglycerides, pancreatitis, liver disease, or congestive heart failure, drinking even moderate amounts of alcohol may worsen your condition. Also, if you take aspirin regularly for heart health, you want to slow down on the drinking. Talk to your health care provider to see what's right for you.

# *Looking at the Mediterranean Diet's Effect on Heart Disease*

The Mediterranean diet is most noticed in the scientific community for its effect on heart health. Heart disease is the number one cause of death in the United States, even though a few lifestyle changes make it easily preventable. Genetics still play a strong role, of course, but making small changes to your diet and exercising make a big difference.

The first research focused on the Mediterranean diet started with a scientist named Ancel Keys and the Seven Countries Study. This study found that southern Europe had far fewer coronary deaths than northern Europe and the United States did, even when factoring in age, smoking, blood pressure, and physical activity. These results made researchers look more closely at the differences in dietary habits. This study is still important today because more people in the Mediterranean regions studied no longer eat in their traditional way, and those regions show higher occurrences of heart disease.

Recent research continues to show a correlation between a traditional Mediterranean diet and lower incidence of heart disease. According to a 2008 study published in the *British Medical Journal,* research showed a 9 percent decrease in deaths from coronary artery disease. A 2011 review of several studies covering 535,000 people that was published in the *Journal of the American College of Cardiology* reported that a traditional Mediterranean diet is associated with lower blood pressure, blood sugar, and triglyceride levels.

In 2013, the *New England Journal of Medicine*'s website published results of a study of 7,447 participants who were randomly assigned to one of three groups: one that followed a Mediterranean diet and supplemented with olive oil; one that followed a Mediterranean diet and supplemented with nuts; and one that was supposed to follow a lowfat diet. All study participants were demonstrated to be at high risk of having cardiovascular problems. The study was ended early (after about five years) because its results indicated that eating the traditional Mediterranean diet substantially reduced the risk of heart attack, stroke, and heart disease–related death among this high-risk population.

# Fighting Cancer

Another area of research on the Mediterranean diet is the diet's effects on preventing and managing cancer. Specific staples of the diet have been shown to provide cancer-preventing and cancer-fighting benefits:

- ✔ **Plant foods:** A diet high in plant foods such as fruits, vegetables, legumes, and nuts may provide cancer protection. The high amounts of phytochemicals in these foods provide unique properties that can help inhibit or slow tumor growth or simply protect your cells. Head to the earlier section "Eating colorfully to get phytochemicals" for details on these powerhouses.

- ✔ **Meat:** Beginning in 1976, researchers from the Harvard School of Public Health followed 88,000 healthy women and found that the risk of colon cancer was 2.5 times higher in women who ate beef, pork, or lamb daily compared with those who ate those meats once a month or less. They also found that the risk of getting colon cancer was directly correlated to the amount of meat eaten.

> ✔ **Olive oil:** A study of 26,000 Greek people pub-
> lished in the *British Journal of Cancer* showed
> that using more olive oil cut cancer risk by 9
> percent.

In addition to these ingredient-specific studies, the
diet as a whole has some promising research. A 2008
study review published in the *British Medical Journal*
showed that following a traditional Mediterranean
diet reduced the risk of dying from cancer by 9 percent. That same year, the *American Journal of Clinical
Nutrition* published a study that showed that among
post-menopausal women, those who followed a traditional Mediterranean diet were 22 percent less likely
to develop breast cancer. Although more research is
needed in this area, you can enjoy a Mediterranean
diet and know that you're helping increase your odds
against cancer.

# Battling Diabetes

The foods in a Mediterranean diet make perfect sense
for a person with type 2 diabetes because the food
choices lean toward being low-glycemic. The *glycemic
index* is a measurement given to carbohydrate-
containing foods that shows how quickly they turn
into blood sugar. High-glycemic foods create a quick,
high blood sugar spike, while low-glycemic foods offer
a slow blood sugar rise.

A diet that provides a slow rise in blood sugar is best
for diabetics, who can't manage a large influx of sugar
normally. Most vegetables, fruits, whole grains, and
legumes (hallmarks of the Mediterranean diet) provide a much slower blood sugar response compared
to white bread, white pasta, or sugary snacks. A 2009
study from the Second University of Naples in Italy,
published in the *Annals of Internal Medicine*, found
that diabetics who followed a Mediterranean diet

instead of a lowfat diet had better glycemic control and were less likely to need diabetes medication.

The portion sizes in the Mediterranean diet can also make a significant difference for a diabetic. Starchy foods such as the whole grains found in cereals and breads can also make blood sugar rise if a person consumes too much of them, but the portion sizes associated with a Mediterranean pattern of eating are much lower and help keep total carbohydrate intake during the meal in check.

# Coffee's health benefits: Full of beans?

The art of drinking coffee was invented by the Italians and has held a strong tradition in many cultures. Coffee is a complex nutrition topic because it's a natural, plant-based food containing healthy antioxidants, which may be to thank for the lower rates of type 2 diabetes, Parkinson's disease, and dementia in coffee drinkers. However, the caffeine in coffee may increase blood pressure (though you can drink decaf to avoid this problem), and coffee in general may increase homocysteine levels, which is a risk factor for heart disease, regardless of the caffeine content. More research is needed to provide any definitive recommendations for or against caffeine and coffee, but enjoying it in moderation is likely the key.

Enjoying *espresso,* a form of concentrated coffee, is a tradition on the Mediterranean coast, but folks there tend to look at espresso as a morning drink only and often drink just one to two ounces of espresso a day (a stark contrast to many coffee-shop regulars in the United States). One ounce of espresso contains around 75 milligrams of caffeine, compared to 135 milligrams in one cup of coffee.

If you don't drink coffee, there is certainly no reason for you to start. If you're a coffee lover, enjoy your coffee, but try to limit yourself to one to two 8-ounce cups of coffee or one to two 1-ounce shots of espresso each day.

But the benefits aren't exclusive to people who already have diabetes; this diet pattern may help you reduce your risk of getting the disease. The SUN cohort study from the University of Navarro, Spain, which involved more than 13,000 participants with no history of diabetes, showed that those participants who followed a Mediterranean-style diet were less likely to develop type 2 diabetes. What's more interesting about this study is that participants who had high risk factors for type 2 diabetes (including older age, family history of diabetes, and a history of smoking) and followed the diet pattern strictly had an 83 percent relative reduction for developing the disease.

# Aging Gracefully: Anti-Aging Tips from the Mediterranean

A Mediterranean lifestyle can also help you feel and look your best. A diet high in nutrients, moderate activity, and lots of laughter with friends lets you enjoy the benefits of health! Here are some of the ways you can age gracefully with a Mediterranean lifestyle.

- ✔ **Increased longevity:** The NIH-AARP Diet and Health Study published in the *Archives of Internal Medicine* in 2007 found that people who closely adhered to a Mediterranean-style diet were 12 to 20 percent less likely to die from cancer and all causes.

- ✔ **Wrinkle reduction:** Now we know we've got your attention! A study published in the *Journal of the American College of Nutrition* in 2001 found that people who consumed a diet high in fruits, vegetables, nuts, legumes, and fish had less skin wrinkling. Of course, this arena needs far more research, but try the theory out at home to see your own results. Sure beats plastic surgery, right?

✔ **Smoother skin:** Eating a diet high in vitamin C foods, such as oranges, strawberries, and broccoli, plays an important role in the production of collagen, the skin's support structure. Head to the section "Fighting free radicals with antioxidants" earlier in the chapter for more vitamin C-rich foods.

✔ **Bone density maintenance:** Moderate weight-bearing exercise such as walking or lifting weights can maintain good bone density, keeping your bones strong and helping you avoid bone fractures later in life.

✔ **Tension taming:** A good laugh reduces tension and stress in the body, leaving your muscles relaxed for up to 45 minutes. Stress can lead to depression, anxiety, high blood pressure, and heart disease, all of which contribute to aging and a reduced quality of life.

✔ **Inflammation reduction:** Inflammation can affect your heart health, joints, and skin. Eating a diet high in anti-inflammatory foods such as cold-water fish, walnuts, flaxseeds, and fresh herbs can help keep you feeling your best.

✔ **Lowered Alzheimer's risk:** A 2006 study at Columbia University Medical Center showed that participants who followed a Mediterranean-style diet had a 40 percent lower risk of Alzheimer's disease than those who didn't.

# Chapter 3

# Losing Weight with the Mediterranean Diet

*Y*ou may be looking for a way to lose some weight and think that the Mediterranean diet is the way to go. Choosing a Mediterranean diet isn't going to be a traditional "diet" or a quick fix. Rather, it's a series of healthy lifestyle choices that can get you to your weight loss goal while you eat delicious, flavorful foods and get out and enjoy life. Sounds much better than counting calories and depriving yourself, right?

With that description in mind, you need to focus on a few must-haves with the Mediterranean lifestyle in order to lose weight successfully. You have to pay attention to lifestyle changes, manage your calorie intake through balancing food choices and controlling portions, and increase your physical activity. This chapter covers all these topics.

# Focusing on Lifestyle Changes

The focus of the Mediterranean diet is on your entire lifestyle. Paying attention to lifestyle changes, such as changing your portion sizes and exercising regularly, is the only way to see long-term results. Weight-loss diets come and go, and most can help you lose the weight, but they aren't something you can live with long term. The Mediterranean diet helps you pay attention to your individual lifestyle, including the types of foods you eat, the portion sizes you consume, your physical activities, and your overall way of life. You can incorporate these changes into your daily life and create long-term habits that bring you not only weight loss but also sustained weight loss.

Evaluating your life and deciding what types of changes will work for you long term is crucial. You want to incorporate changes you're excited to make; if you feel like you *have* to make them, you may struggle to motivate yourself and find that you keep pushing the changes off for another day. Making changes that work for you sets the stage so that you can keep the weight off long term.

The following sections focus on the main lifestyle changes you can make by integrating the Mediterranean diet into your daily life. These changes include setting goals, such as slowing down and making time for yourself, and quitting quick-fix diets. After you commit to focusing on lifestyle changes, remember to start small with baby steps.

## Setting goals

Making goals provides a road map of where you are so that you're less likely to get lost in the details of lifestyle changes. In order for your goals to be attainable, they must be realistic, practical, and measureable:

- ✔ **Realistic goals:** Make sure your goals are realistic ones that you can successfully achieve. For example, if you have 50 pounds to lose, don't set a goal to lose all the weight in two months. This unrealistic timeline may make you frustrated and inclined to give up if you don't hit that mark.

- ✔ **Practical goals:** What's "practical" depends entirely on your lifestyle. If your day is scheduled around traveling from place to place, setting a goal of eating lunch at home may not be practical. Instead, you can make a goal to bring a healthy lunch or have a deli sandwich and salad instead of buzzing through a fast-food joint for a grease-bomb combo (hold the tomato).

- ✔ **Measurable goals:** You won't know whether you're meeting your goals if you can't measure them. Specific goals, such as eating three servings of vegetables per day, are a lot easier to measure than general goals such as "eat healthy."

## Ditching diets

Quitting diets is the first step to weight-loss success. Chronic dieting ends up doing more harm than good. If you've lost weight and regained it many times, you may have noticed how easy it is to gain. Each time you lose and gain weight, you may be lowering your *metabolic rate* (how many calories your body burns at rest), making gaining weight easier and easier; any time you consume more calories than you burn, you gain weight. The biggest issue with traditional dieting is that it almost always provides a short-term solution.

Omitting foods, counting calories, and eating very low numbers of calories aren't habits most people can live with long term. You may lose weight quickly with these kinds of methods, but you'll likely gain it back (plus possibly even more weight) after you stop the diet, leaving you in a never-ending battle with weight loss that affects your self-esteem and motivation.

Dieting also messes with your head. Research shows that when people restrict and omit foods, they tend to focus more on those foods, which leads to an unhealthy relationship. For example, when you say you aren't going to eat any sugar, you're more likely to dwell on chocolate, ice cream, and other forbidden goodies until you snap and end up eating more of the items than you should. Then you say, "I'll get back on track next week," and the cycle continues and continues.

Assuming you have no health issues that require you to omit certain foods, research shows that enjoying a small piece of, say, chocolate and then moving on is better for you than omitting sugar altogether. You don't become consumed with the chocolate and are less likely to overeat it. Finding the balance of eating healthy foods most of the time and allowing yourself treats once in a while is key to mastering weight loss.

## *Making time in a fast-paced world*

A fast-paced lifestyle is part of reality today, but it also contradicts one of the premises of a Mediterranean lifestyle. When incorporating the Mediterranean diet into your lifestyle, your first goal is to try to slow down. Look at all you have on your (figurative) plate and see whether you can start to say "no" to some things so you can free up time for yourself.

Overbooking yourself with work, kids, and other tasks is easy. Before you know it, you have no time for health and wellness, leading to overwhelm and fatigue. Children, family, certain occupations, and other obligations may make slowing down more diffi-cult. However, you still can do a few things to make adopting the Mediterranean lifestyle easier. Keep the following tips in mind:

- ✔ **Have a plan for your weekly grocery shopping and meal planning.** Doing so can save you time and help you to follow through with your food goals. See Chapter 4 for ideas to get started.

- ✔ **Pre-make meals and meal components to have at the ready.** Use batch cooking to make meals ahead of time for later in the week or for freez-ing. Chop up a bunch of fresh veggies and pre-pare some simple grains like rice, quinoa, or barley at the beginning of the week to have on hand throughout the week so you can cut down your cooking time after your busy day.

- ✔ **Follow the great Mediterranean strategy of using fresh, raw produce with your meals.** Sometimes cooking all meal components takes up too much time. Add unadorned veggies such as sliced tomatoes and cucumbers or carrot sticks to your plate. Focus on easy-to-prepare meals for every day and use the more labor-intensive cooking for special occasions.

- ✔ **Embrace the convenience of the produce aisle.** Make use of pre-washed, pre-cut vegetables you find at your grocery store, such as salad mixes, baby carrots, grape tomatoes, and celery sticks.

- ✔ **Keep your kitchen well stocked.** That way, you always have Mediterranean foods such as olive oil and beans on hand for throwing together whatever meal strikes your fancy. Chapter 4 runs down some key items you likely want to keep on hand.

✔ **Schedule time for physical activity.** Find 20 to 30 minutes for walking or doing other kinds of exercise four to five times a week and pencil it into your schedule. Make sure you stick to your schedule. Do you tend to watch mindless TV for an hour each evening? If so, reduce your TV time and go walking for 30 minutes. Do you take an hour lunch at work? Go outside and walk for 20 to 30 minutes before you eat.

## *Creating small changes that stick*

Before you begin your weight-loss journey, you want to take baby steps and start small with a few changes at a time. Set small goals that you can integrate into your daily life.

For example, perhaps you start by making sure you have a fruit or vegetable with every meal while decreasing your portions of meats and starch. Add a scheduled daily walk to that goal, and you have a great starting point for incorporating changes. Master these few things, and you'll likely lose a few pounds from your new, lower calorie intake and increase in calorie-burning exercise. A little success is a great way to make changes become habits. Then you're on to the next two goals.

Trying to jump into all the new changes at once can be overwhelming and seem impossible, making you quit before you get a chance to really get rolling. Change can be hard, and your mind will keep calling you back to your old habits. Tackling some small, achievable goals and having a few victories can keep you motivated for the long haul. Even a few small changes each week can lead to weight loss.

# *Considering Calories without Counting Them*

*Calories* are the amount of energy in the foods you eat and the amount of energy your body uses for daily activities. Your body constantly needs energy or fuel not only for daily activities such as cooking, cleaning, and exercising but also for basic biological functions (like breathing). Everyone has a different metabolic rate that determines how quickly he or she burns calories and depends on factors such as age, genetics, gender, and physical fitness level.

You can't lose weight if you eat more calories than you burn through daily activity and exercise. To lose weight, you have to create a calorie deficit, but you can do so without actually knowing how many calories you burn. All you have to do is make small changes to your lifestyle, such as reducing portion sizes and exercising more, to reduce your calorie intake.

Counting the calorie level of each and every food and drink you consume isn't much fun; very few people can do it for the long term. Without having some idea of your calorie intake level, however, you'll be in the dark about how much you're eating. That's where the Mediterranean diet comes into play. Instead of counting calories, you think about the kinds of foods you eat and the portion sizes of those foods. By adding more low-calorie fruits and vegetables to your diet and decreasing the portion size of higher-calorie foods like meats and grains, you can decrease your calorie level naturally. When you master this new way of eating, you can ensure you're eating the appropriate number of calories without having to account for every single one.

The following sections show you how to eat at an appropriate calorie level by properly balancing your plate's food make-up, controlling portions, and expending energy through fun activities.

## Eating more to lose weight

Unlike many weight-loss diets, a Mediterranean style of eating lets you have more food on your plate while still taking in fewer calories. "How does *that* work?" you wonder. Well, you get to eat far more low-calorie vegetables and fewer high-calorie meats and grains. As an added bonus, these lower-calorie foods also help you feel more satisfied with your meal instead of feeling deprived.

In the United States, a traditional plate of food has a large piece of meat, a large serving of grains or potatoes, and a tiny amount of vegetable. By simply switching up your plate to include small portions of meat and grain, two to three vegetables, and perhaps a serving of legumes, you can easily save calories (in some cases, hundreds of them). For example, one 6-ounce chicken breast is around 276 calories. Decrease the serving size to 3 ounces, and the count drops to 138 calories. That one change saves 138 calories. A serving of vegetables (½ cup cooked or 1 cup raw) is only 25 calories. By the time you put two to three of those servings on your plate, you've spent about 75 calories and don't have space for much else. You can see how simply changing the balance of the foods you eat makes a huge difference in your calorie intake.

## Taking portion size into account

Paying attention to portion sizes is a far better way to decrease your calorie intake than counting calories. Portion sizes in the Mediterranean are different than they are in the United States, which is one reason folks in the Mediterranean region tend to manage their weights more effectively. Although the U.S. serving-size guidelines are appropriate, few Americans actually follow them.

Part of the problem is that the portion sizes in restaurants have become gigantic — big enough to feed three adults in some circumstances. Even the plate sizes are huge! The more you see restaurant portion sizes, the more normal they seem.

On the Mediterranean coast, people actually eat portion sizes of meats and grains closer to what the recommended serving sizes are in the United States: 2 to 3 ounces of meat as a side dish (recommended U.S. serving: 3 ounces) and about ½ cup of grains/pasta as a side dish (recommended U.S. serving: the same). Unfortunately, the average American is eating closer to 8 ounces of meat and 1½ to 2 cups of grains at any given meal. Table 3-1 is a serving guide that can help you create smaller, appropriate portions and thus a lower-calorie plate; after you get the hang of it, eating the right portion size will be second nature, and you'll just know how much to put on your plate by eyeballing it.

| Table 3-1 | Serving Size Guide |
|-----------|---------------------|
| **Food** | **Serving Size** |
| Grains | 1 slice bread |
| | ½ an English muffin, hamburger bun, or bagel |
| | ⅓ cup rice |
| | ½ cup cooked cereal, pasta, or other cooked grain |
| | ¾ cup cold cereal |
| | One 6-inch tortilla |

*(continued)*

## Table 3-1 *(continued)*

| Food | Serving Size |
| --- | --- |
| Other starchy carbohydrates | ½ cup beans or lentils (these also contain protein) |
| Fruit | 1 medium piece of fruit |
| | ½ cup canned or sliced fruit |
| | 6 ounces (¾ cup) 100% fruit juice |
| Vegetables | 1 cup raw |
| | ½ cup cooked |
| | 6 ounces (¾ cup) 100% vegetable juice |
| Dairy | 8 ounces of milk or yogurt |
| | ⅓ cup cottage cheese |
| | 1 ounce cheese |
| Protein | ½ cup beans (beans are also high in carbs) |
| | 2–4 ounces beef, poultry, pork, or fish (size of a deck of cards) |
| | 1 ounce cheese |
| | 1 egg |
| | 1 ounce nuts |
| | 1 tablespoon nut spreads (such as peanut butter, almond butter, and so on) |
| Fats | ⅛ of an avocado (2 tablespoons) |
| | 1 teaspoon oil, butter, margarine, or mayonnaise |
| | 2 teaspoons whipped butter |
| | 8 olives |
| | 1 tablespoon regular salad dressing |
| | 2 tablespoons lowfat salad dressing |

Here's an example of what a Mediterranean style meal may look like using these serving sizes.

- ✔ 2 ounces of grilled lemon chicken

- ✔ ⅔ cup of wild rice, black bean, and fresh herb mixture

- ✔ 2 cups of mixed green salad with sliced tomatoes and radishes with 1 tablespoon vinaigrette salad dressing

- ✔ ½ cup grilled zucchini

This large meal contains several vegetable servings, and the estimated calorie level is about 500 calories. Compare that to an 8-ounce chicken breast with 2 cups of rice and a small vegetable; that calorie level is about 680 calories. This sample Mediterranean meal isn't too bad when you consider that you get to eat a greater variety of food, a good balance of protein between the chicken and black beans, and loads of fiber from the beans and veggies to help you feel full and satisfied. It also contains a good dose of healthy fats from the salad dressing and any oil used while grilling the zucchini.

## *Watching your fat calories*

The Mediterranean diet also allows you to keep track of the calories you get from fat. Although people on the Mediterranean coast eat slightly more fat than is recommended in the United States (35 percent of their calories come from fat, versus the U.S. recommendation of 30 percent), they consume different types of fats, such as the healthy fats from olive oil. Flip to Chapter 2 for details on the types of fat you consume on a Mediterranean diet.

No matter what type of fat you eat, it still has 9 calories per gram. Make sure you're careful about not using too much fat with your meals. Otherwise, you can end up gaining weight from excessive fat calories.

To help you gauge how much fat to use in your cooking, measure your added fats, such as salad dressing or drizzles of olive oil, for a few days so that you get the idea of what the appropriate portion size looks like on your food. You want to use about one tablespoon of salad dressing and one teaspoon for oil drizzles added to vegetables or breads. You don't need to measure forever, and you don't need to be exact. Just get comfortable with the portion, and pretty soon you'll be able to eye what a teaspoon of oil looks like.

## *Increasing activity you love*

Exercise is an important component to weight loss and health; you have to use up some of your calorie intake as energy, or those calories will store as fat. Exercise allows you to burn calories and to strengthen your heart, manage stress, and increase your energy level.

Starting an exercise program may be challenging for you — maybe the thought of going to a busy gym and running on a treadmill sounds more painful than a double root canal. Never fear; look to the Mediterranean. On the Mediterranean coast, people tend to get exercise by walking, working, and doing enjoyable activities instead of through formalized exercise programs. That is, people walk to run errands; lift and carry groceries home; work in the yard; and enjoy fun activities like bike riding or swimming.

If starting an exercise program sounds difficult for you, find activities that you actually enjoy doing and look for ways to get out every day for a walk. The American College of Sports Medicine and the American Heart Association recommend getting 30 minutes of moderate exercise (you get your heart rate up but can still have a conversation) a day, five days a week for those who are 18 to 65 years old, as well as adding two days a week of strength-training exercises like lifting weights.

# Suppressing Your Appetite Naturally

Eating a Mediterranean-style diet is not only great for your health but can also work as a natural appetite suppressant to help manage your weight. When you eat the right balance of plant-based foods and healthy fats, your body works in a natural way to feel satisfied. Because you're full, you're not tempted (at least, not by your stomach) to snack on high-calorie junk food a short while after your last meal. The following sections highlight the three main reasons a Mediterranean diet helps to control your appetite.

## Loading up on fiber

Fiber, found in fruits, vegetables, whole grains, and legumes, provides bulk and slows down digestion to help you feel full for a longer period of time. With the Mediterranean diet, you consume much more fiber-rich food with each meal and snack, which can make you feel satisfied all day. The average American diet contains little fiber and often doesn't include fibrous foods with each meal; this lack of fiber can actually stimulate your appetite even shortly after you've eaten.

High-fiber foods also make you chew a little longer, helping you to slow down at mealtime. Your brain takes 20 minutes to register that you're full, which is longer than many people spend eating a meal. As a result, your brain may give you the okay to keep eating because it doesn't realize yet that you've actually eaten enough to be full. Chewing more helps you to slow down and reach that 20-minute mark.

## *Turning on your fullness hormones*

The Mediterranean diet is naturally high in *low-glycemic foods,* those carbohydrate-containing foods that illicit a lower blood sugar spike. Low-glycemic foods may just help kick on your fullness response. Appetite is controlled by an intricate dance of hormones that trigger the feelings of hunger and fullness.

When you're eating, your body releases two separate hormones that play a role in regulating your appetite and letting you know you're full. Those hormones are

✔ **Leptin:** This hormone releases a process telling you it's time to stop eating — you're comfortably full.

✔ **GLP-1:** This hormone tells your body, "Hey, I'm not messing around. You need to stop eating pronto because the food is making you uncomfortably full." It brings things to a halt by telling your stomach to stop moving anything along to your intestines until they've broken down what's already there. You know how after you eat a huge meal like Thanksgiving dinner, all you can do is lie on the couch in sweatpants? That's your GLP-1 kicking in.

In 2009, researchers from King's College in London took a close look at GLP-1 in respect to a low-glycemic diet. Volunteers who ate a low-glycemic breakfast ended up with 20 percent higher levels of GLP-1 in their blood compared to those who ate a high-glycemic breakfast.

More research is needed, but as you start eating the Mediterranean way, you can take note of whether you feel a larger degree of fullness after your meals than you have in the past.

To help you pay attention to your body, start by filling your plate with appropriate portion sizes of food (see the serving size guide in Table 3-1). Eat slowly, spending at least 20 minutes with your meal. Keep checking in with your stomach and pay attention to whether it feels hungry, neutral, or full. You'll be surprised that a relatively small amount of food will make you feel comfortably full. At this point, you want to stop eating.

Feeling biologically full and psychologically satisfied with your meal are two very different things that are often hard to distinguish. Biological fullness occurs in your stomach, where you feel hungry, neutral, or comfortably full. Feeling psychologically satisfied is in your brain; you want to eat more because it tastes so good!

Overindulging once in a while because something is so tasty is completely normal, but when you consistently ignore your fullness cues and eat until you're psychologically satisfied, you consume too many calories far too often. If you fall into this trap, tell yourself you can have more of the food later in the day or even tomorrow. Heck, you can even make this meal again and again so that you can enjoy it every week.

*Note:* One of the first signs of dehydration is hunger, so when you feel hungry even though you just ate a short time ago, grab a glass of water, wait 15 minutes, and see how you feel.

# Controlling Food Cravings

Food cravings occur for many reasons, whether they're physiological, psychological, or a combination of both. For instance, having a stressful day at work may lead to food cravings. Perhaps you end up skipping a meal (putting more stress on your body) and start craving some particular candy that was your go-to feel-better solution growing up. At this point, eating that candy is easy, even if you have an apple sitting in your drawer.

Unfortunately, no one-size-fits-all-answer exists to deal with food cravings, but you can do a few things to manage them more effectively. The following strategies are natural byproducts of a Mediterranean style of living.

## Avoiding blood sugar spikes

Keeping your blood sugar stable throughout the day is a good strategy to help manage food cravings. Eating high-glycemic foods causes a high blood sugar spike and then a crash, leaving you with symptoms of low blood sugar that include hunger and irritability, which can lead down the path to food cravings. Waiting too long to eat between meals and snacks can also elicit those low blood sugar symptoms. The combination of feeling both very hungry and edgy can often set you up to make the wrong food choices.

 To avoid this trap, do as they do on the Mediterranean coast, including the following:

✔ **Make sure you don't skip meals or wait longer than 5 hours to eat.** Eat a meal or snack every 3 to 5 hours. Eat when you are hungry instead of waiting until you have extreme hunger.

✔ **Eat protein-rich foods and a bit of fat.** Include foods such as fish, beans, nuts, or eggs with a fat with each meal to help slow down your digestion.

✔ **Eat high fiber fruits, vegetables, grains, and legumes with each meal and snack.** You don't have to eat these foods all at once, but including some combination of them at meals and incorporating a fruit, veggie, or whole grain with your snacks is a good idea.

## Managing your stress hormones

Stress occurs for many different reasons, and unfortunately, it's a prevalent part of everyday life for many people. You may have a demanding job and small children to care for. Perhaps the lack of time to stick to a proper diet and exercise plan is stressful. Luckily, the Mediterranean lifestyle can help you handle your stress and find a little bit of relaxation.

Stress releases hormones that trigger the "fight or flight" response (where your body gears up its energy levels for a big event like fighting or fleeing) and kick on your hunger hormones. Biologically, this concept makes sense. How are you supposed to fight like a warrior or run to the hills with no fuel? The body is working as it's supposed to. The increase in stress is what's leading to more hunger and food cravings.

 You can tackle stress-induced cravings a few different ways:

✔ **Try to limit or prevent stressful situations in your life.** Some things you can't help, like work-related stress, but you can certainly prevent stress in other ways, like saying "no" more often if you have too much going on or avoiding unnecessary confrontations by letting the small stuff in life go.

✔ **Manage stress levels.** This step is a priority in traditional Mediterranean life. You can accomplish it by exercising, getting enough sleep, drinking water, practicing deep breathing, meditating, and relaxing. For example, if you are getting ready for a stressful meeting, take a few moments to do some deep breathing. Simply take a deep breath, hold it for a few seconds, and let the air out. Keep repeating for as long as you can. Even a few minutes can help.

✔ **When you're feeling a craving, go for a low-glycemic snack and include some omega-3 fatty acids.** A good snack is some tuna fish spread on whole-grain crackers. This combination can help you get the fuel your body is craving but also help your central nervous system calm down. Eating high-glycemic foods in this situation can keep you in a state of blood sugar spikes, making the craving cycle worse.

✔ **Know when to give in a little.** If you're really craving sugar, are in a truly edgy state, and couldn't care less about what you *should* eat, eat the omega-3 and low-glycemic snack and then have a small piece of the sugar you're craving. The healthy snack will do its work biologically, and the small sugar hit will help you avoid feeling deprived to the point where you want to eat the whole package.

These tips may require changing your coping habits. Your brain may be used to going for comfort food when you're stressed, so you need to go through a period of retraining your brain to try some new coping skills, such as having a cup of tea and journaling for a few minutes to help come down from the stressful day.

# *Mastering the Art of Mindful Eating*

A traditional Mediterranean style of eating engages regularly in mindful eating, something that many people have completely lost track of. With *mindful eating,* you can manage your weight by paying attention to your internal body cues. Yes, your own body has a very sophisticated weight management system built in that include hormones that tell you when you should eat and when to stop (see the earlier section "Suppressing Your Appetite Naturally" for details). The problem is that too many people often ignore that reflex. The following sections highlight how to refocus on these internal cues and become completely satisfied with what you're eating.

## *Slowing down*

Slowing down is a theme in the Mediterranean lifestyle that even goes for meals. A good goal is to spend at least 20 to 30 minutes eating your larger meals. As we note earlier in the chapter, this time frame gives your biological system time to let you know when you're full. Plus, it allows you to sit and enjoy your food. Use these tips to help you slow down at meal time:

- ✔ Set your fork down between bites.
- ✔ Take a deep breath and count to ten before each bite.
- ✔ Have great table discussions with your family and friends. Ask a question about everyone's day or talk about current events.
- ✔ Make meal time a television-, computer-, and phone-free zone to avoid mindless eating.

## *Enjoying food to its fullest*

When you eat, take time to enjoy every aspect of your food. When you think about Italians, Greeks, Spaniards, and other Mediterranean people, you think about cultures who love their food. This enjoyment of food helps them to manage their weights by feeling psychologically satisfied with what they're eating, which leaves less chance for overeating.

Incorporate the following mealtime tips to help you enjoy eating to the fullest:

✔ **Take a deep breath.** Before you dig into any food, smell the flavors coming from it.

✔ **Act like the natives.** Put yourself in the shoes of an Italian or Greek when you're eating a meal and rave over every bite.

✔ **Taste each and every flavor.** During each bite, let the food sit in your mouth. Chew it slowly and take pleasure in the freshness and the many tastes that roll across your taste buds. By slowing down and really tasting the flavors, you'll be more satisfied than you would be eating it quickly. Don't underestimate the power of food satisfaction. Not being satisfied with what you're eating can lead to overeating relatively easily.

Additionally, serving lots of food in small portion sizes helps you enjoy each flavor. Adding several vegetables, sliced tomatoes, olives, salads, and protein to a meal helps you to enjoy all the different flavors and temperatures.

You can do the chocolate kiss test at home to see for yourself how luxuriating in your food makes you eat less. Take a chocolate kiss and wolf it down quickly. How did it taste? Would you be able to report to someone about the texture and flavor? Wouldn't it be easy to pop another couple in your mouth considering how quickly that went? Now, try again, and let the candy melt in your mouth for as long as you can. No chewing; just slowly melt it. You can see how you're more satisfied with the flavor and need less food to get you to that psychological satisfaction level.

## Maximizing Your Metabolic Rate

Your metabolic rate is how many calories you burn at rest. You don't have control over some of the factors that influence this rate, but you can take some steps to kick your metabolic rate into full gear. Incorporate some of these strategies in your daily living; try to include at least two to three of these strategies regularly:

- ✔ **Build lean muscle mass.** Muscle burns 90 percent more calories than fat does, so the more muscle you have, the more calories you burn each day. You can build more muscle by lifting weights, using resistance bands, walking, and performing other forms of strength-training exercises.

- ✔ **Increase your heart rate.** Regular aerobic exercise not only gets your heart rate up but also raises your metabolism during the activity and for several hours afterwards. Aerobic exercise includes any activity that gets your heart rate up, such as walking, biking, dancing, jogging, swimming, or aerobics classes.

- ✔ **Take the extra stairs.** Any time you increase your heart rate, even for two minutes, you give your metabolic rate a small boost. So doing little things all day like taking the stairs, dancing to your favorite song, or walking farther in the parking lot provides little rises in your metabolic rate over the course of a day. Those little individual rises add up to help you with weight loss and wellness. As you move through your day, think of ways you can increase these little bursts of energy.

✔ **Enjoy some resistant starches.** Research shows a connection between metabolism and certain starch-resistant foods that can increase the body's efficiency at burning stored fat. *Resistant starch* refers to a type of fiber that opposes digestion. Unlike other types of fiber, resistant starch ferments in the large intestine, which creates beneficial fatty acids, including one called *butyrate.*

This particular fatty acid has been shown to help the body burn more stored fat. You can find resistant starches in bananas, yams, pearl barley, and corn — all pieces of a Mediterranean-style diet. The only trick is to eat these foods cold or at room temperature for their best effect, and remember that they're not a miracle cure.

# Chapter 4

# Planning, Shopping, and Cooking for Success

- - - - - - - - - - - - - - - - - - - - - - - - - -

## *In This Chapter*

▶ Building meals with a Mediterranean mindset

▶ Stocking your pantry, fridge, and freezer

▶ Adopting some new cooking habits

- - - - - - - - - - - - - - - - - - - - - - - - - -

*L*iving the Mediterranean lifestyle requires giving some advance thought to what you're going to eat, stocking your kitchen with the staples you need to create healthy meals, and adjusting your cooking habits. Preparing food at home rather than relying on restaurants and convenience foods is certainly a huge part of moving toward a Mediterranean lifestyle.

In this chapter, we offer suggestions for getting started with meal planning, shopping for Mediterranean staples, and making a couple easy and essential changes in your cooking habits.

# Grasping the Importance of Meal Planning

Meal planning provides you a road map for the week of what you're going to eat, when you'll prepare those meals, and what foods you need to have handy in your kitchen to do so. If you tend to eat at restaurants because of your work situation or other schedule demands, meal planning can also involve preparing yourself to make better choices when perusing a menu. By taking the steps to do some planning, changing to a Mediterranean diet is much easier and less stressful.

Meal planning on some level is important for several reasons:

- ✔ It ensures that you're efficient with your time and have everything you need on hand.

- ✔ It makes cooking easier during the week because you already know what you're making instead of trying to think of what you can cook with the chicken and cauliflower you bought.

- ✔ It saves you money by decreasing food waste.

- ✔ It helps you fight temptation when you're in a restaurant facing a menu full of heavy, cream-laden, or otherwise not heart-healthy dishes.

## Picking a planning approach

Meal planning needs to (and can) work into your life-style. Here are a few different approaches; try to find one that works for you:

✔ **The detailed meal plan:** Sit down and write out a plan for breakfast, lunch, and dinner for each day of the week. (You may want to include snacks as well.) You can make each day's foods interchangeable, but this method at least makes sure you have a plan and can go on your way this week with everything organized.

✔ **The rotating two-week meal plan:** Spend some time making up a two-week meal plan, complete with shopping list, and you've done all the work you need. So it may be that you have scrambled eggs with dill every other Monday for breakfast and tortellini with vegetables and pesto every other Sunday for dinner. You still get plenty of variety with a two-week meal plan, but you may need to change it up every couple of months to make seasonal menus.

✔ **The fast meal plan:** If you're like author Meri, you don't want to waste time on making a meal plan for each and every meal for the week. In that case, think about your habits and plan accordingly. For example, Meri knows she regularly eats a few different items for breakfast, such as poached eggs or granola and yogurt, and often eats leftovers or sandwiches along with fruit for lunch. So she focuses only on planning dinners and the few staples she needs for breakfast and lunch. She also doesn't plan a meal every night because her family almost always uses leftovers as another meal. Making a menu plan for four to five nights a week works out just fine for her situation.

✔ **The super-fast meal plan:** Perhaps you need something even speedier than the fast menu plan. Instead of planning four or five dinners a week, focus on two to three and plan some convenience meals, such as entree salads you can throw together or canned or homemade, frozen soups.

## *Changing the way you fill your plate*

Folks on the Mediterranean coast eat many of the same foods that people elsewhere do; they just eat smaller portions and incorporate plenty of vegetables. For example, they may eat pizza, but they eat less pizza; go easy on the sauce, cheese, and other toppings; and add a salad and possibly other side vegetables. In this section, we highlight some of the Mediterranean eating habits you can adopt when you're meal planning. These small changes make all the difference in health — as well as in flavor.

### *Focusing on plant-based foods*

To get more plant-based foods on your plate, plan to include one to two fruits and/or veggies (in a rainbow of colors) in each meal, and use beans or lentils as your protein several times a week. Meats and starchy carbohydrates become your side dishes. Think about all the fresh flavors of the Mediterranean and try putting some items together. Here are some ideas to get you started:

✔ **Soup and sandwich:** The standby of grilled cheese sandwich and tomato soup is appropriate for lunch or dinner. Why stop at just the tomato soup, though? Consider adding more veggies to the soup, throwing some fresh basil and tomato onto your sandwich, and including a side salad along with your meal.

✔ **Sandwiches:** Pump up your favorite sandwich with tomatoes or cucumbers. If you don't like them in a sandwich, toss them with a little oil and vinegar for a side dish. Add a fruit for a complete meal.

✔ **Salads, salads, salads:** We recommend always having salad greens on hand because they can make a quick side dish or a whole meal. Add as many veggies and fruits as you can find and top with a protein, such as nuts, beans, hard-boiled egg, or leftover chicken or fish. Add a roll or slice of toast, and you have a quick, light meal for a busy evening.

✔ **Rice and beans:** Top brown rice with your favorite beans (try black or pinto), chopped fresh tomatoes, bell peppers, and whatever else you love. Sprinkle with some goat cheese or feta cheese, and you have delicious fast food with lots of fresh produce! For extra flavor, add some fresh herbs such as cilantro or basil.

✔ **Scrambled eggs:** Eggs with a slice of toast can work for any meal of the day. Sauté vegetables such as onions, zucchini, bell peppers, tomatoes, and spinach, and add them to your eggs. Top with a little salsa for some kick!

✔ **Frozen meals:** Some frozen meals are better than others, so try to find some with lower sodium and fat contents and stick to basic foods. Even if your meal contains vegetables, add more as a side dish or to the entree; it's as easy as tossing some grape tomatoes and cucumbers onto your plate.

✔ **Leftovers:** Don't underestimate the power of batch cooking. Consider making extra meal portions (or just extra portions of certain ingredients) and utilizing them later in the week. Maybe you make some extra cooked barley; combine it with some beans and veggies. Have some grilled chicken in the fridge? Slice it up and add it to a salad. Grilled vegetables? Put them in a tortilla with beans and cheese.

### Making good use of healthy fats

Eating Mediterranean cooking doesn't mean you have to go on a lowfat diet. You just focus on different types of fats, tipping the balance toward healthy monounsaturated fat sources such as olive oil, olives, nuts, and avocadoes and away from saturated fats such as animal fats. Using monounsaturated fats is often associated with better heart health. Eating a good amount of dietary fat also helps to keep you feeling full for a longer period of time.

 Here are some tips to add healthy fats in place of not-so-healthy fats when you plan your meals:

✔ Use olive oil rather than vegetable oils or butter when sautéing meats and vegetables.

✔ Use salad dressings with an olive oil base rather than those with a base of cream or other vegetable oils.

✔ When making a grilled sandwich, brush your bread with olive oil rather than butter.

✔ Dip your bread in extra-virgin olive oil and a little balsamic vinegar instead of using butter.

✔ Spread avocado, pesto, or hummus on your sandwiches and use less (or no) mayonnaise.

### Finding the right balance with protein

Many people automatically consider protein foods such as beef, poultry, pork, and fish as an entree. However, meat is typically a side dish in the Mediterranean diet; when meat is served as the main dish, it's in a smaller portion size than you're probably used to.

 The goal is to eat less animal protein and more plant-based protein. Instead of planning to serve an 8-ounce steak for dinner, maybe you serve a 3- or 4-ounce portion but also have a lentil salad or sprinkle some nuts on a salad to reincorporate some of that lost protein.

You don't have to become vegetarian to live a Mediterranean lifestyle. Incorporating this lifestyle is about eating less of the unhealthy stuff and adding more variety to your plate — not about depriving yourself completely.

### *Looking at a Mediterranean meal makeover*

Everyone loves a good makeover story. We want to show you how powerful small changes can be and also emphasize that you don't have to give up foods you love when you plan meals with a Mediterranean mindset.

#### Before: A typical steak-and-potatoes meal

8-ounce rib-eye steak

Whole baked potato with sour cream and butter

½ cup steamed broccoli

*Estimated calories: 1,049; Saturated fat: 22 grams; Monounsaturated fat: 15.8 grams*

#### After: A Mediterranean-style steak-and-potatoes meal

3-ounce rib-eye steak

¾ cup Garlic and Lemon Roasted Potatoes (see Chapter 6 for the recipe)

½ cup steamed broccoli

Grilled fennel

*Estimated calories: 575; Saturated fat: 5 grams; Monounsaturated fat: 26 grams*

Decreasing the amount of steak, changing the (saturated fat) loaded baked potato to the roasted potatoes made using olive oil, and adding more vegetables changed the entire make-up of this meal. The made-over meal has nearly half the calories, significantly lower levels of saturated fats, and much higher levels of healthy monounsaturated fats. Plus, the grilled fennel adds vitamins, minerals, and phytochemicals.

# Getting involved with your local CSA

Buying a share of a Community Supported Agriculture (CSA) is a great way to incorporate fresh, seasonal produce into your diet. With a CSA, you pay an upfront fee to a local farm and receive a box full of fresh produce each week in return. Going with a CSA is as close to having your own garden as you can get without having to get dirt under your fingernails, and it's a great way to get into the Mediterranean style of living. Plus, you support your local farmers.

With the amazing fresh produce you get with a CSA, take time to learn how to cook seasonally. Get into the practice of using what's fresh and available, and plan your meals accordingly. Doing so can be a little different at first (you may not have a trove of recipes ready that utilize that box of kale, broccoli, and beets you just received), but after you get the hang of it, you may never want to go back.

CSA isn't for everyone. If you're very picky with produce and don't enjoy a wide variety, we suggest sticking to the farmers' market or your grocery store so that you can pick just what you want. Otherwise, you can end up with a box full of veggies you don't enjoy, and it can go to waste.

To find a local CSA, ask some of the vendors at your local farmers' market. Many times, those same vendors offer CSAs from their own farms. You can also search www.local harvest.com, or ask at your local Chamber of Commerce.

# *Stocking Mediterranean Staples*

The following sections provide you with a list of food staples to have on hand in your new Mediterranean kitchen so that you can easily prepare convenient meals and healthy snacks any time instead of feeling like you have to run to the grocery store several times a week.

## Loading up your pantry

A well-organized and well-stocked food supply gives you the ability to make more food from scratch when you want to slow down or to throw together fast meals when you're short on time. Here is a good pantry list to get you started:

- ✔ Oils, including olive oil, extra-virgin olive oil, and nonstick cooking spray

- ✔ Seasonings, including salt, sea salt, black pepper, ground cumin, paprika, garlic powder, chili powder, curry powder, ginger, cinnamon, dill, parsley, tarragon, basil, oregano, thyme, rosemary, and your choice of other dry herbs

- ✔ Canned and/or dried beans, such as black beans, pinto beans, or white beans

- ✔ Lentils

- ✔ Canned soups, such as minestrone, vegetable, or tomato

- ✔ Rice, including wild rice and brown rice

- ✔ Pearl barley, quinoa, or bulgur wheat

- ✔ Pasta

- ✔ Oatmeal

- ✔ Cornmeal

## Buying and storing nuts

Nuts are a common staple on the Mediterranean coast, used for snacking as well as in salads, side dishes, and desserts. Nuts are a good source of healthy monounsaturated fats, but those fats can go rancid if you don't store your nuts properly. Use these guidelines when you buy and store nuts:

✔ Buy nuts from local farmers if available, or at stores that have a high *turnover rate* (meaning they sell foods quickly instead of having them sit for long periods), to ensure freshness.

✔ If possible, buy nuts that include a sell-by date to have a better idea of how old they are. (Buying from bins doesn't necessarily mean they're fresher.)

✔ Store nuts in airtight plastic or glass containers.

✔ Avoid keeping nuts near high-odor foods such as garlic because nuts absorb the smell from their surroundings.

✔ Keep shelled nuts at room temperature for up to three months or refrigerated for four months. Store unshelled nuts for four months in the refrigerator and up to eight months in the freezer.

## *Filling your refrigerator*

Here, we note a few basic fridge foods that you want to always have on hand, in addition to whatever fresh, seasonal veggies you plan to use in your meals:

✔ Carton of eggs

✔ Lean deli meats

✔ Feta or goat cheese

✔ Lowfat Greek yogurt

✔ 1 percent milk

✔ Natural nut butter like peanut butter or almond butter

✔ Condiments, such as mustard, Worcestershire sauce, salsas, and mayonnaise

## *Freezing for the future*

Keeping certain frozen foods on hand for recipes simplifies the cooking process. You may find that the following frozen items come in handy:

- ✔ Frozen spinach, cauliflower, broccoli, and other veggies

- ✔ No-sugar-added frozen fruit such as blueberries (great to thaw out in the morning and add to cereals or oatmeal)

- ✔ Boneless, skinless chicken breasts

- ✔ Fish fillets or salmon burgers

- ✔ Frozen shrimp

## *Filling your countertop*

One of the primary concepts of Mediterranean cooking is having plenty of fresh fruits and vegetables on hand, and having them literally at hand is even better. Many foods, such as tomatoes, lose flavor if you store them in the refrigerator. A good general rule is that if the produce isn't refrigerated at the store, it shouldn't be refrigerated at home.

Here are some fruits and other items that are good to keep at the ready on the counter:

- ✔ Fruits such as apples, oranges, bananas, and pears. Pick your favorites and stock a beautiful fruit bowl on your counter to pick at during the day.

- ✔ Lemons for recipes, to add to your water, or to enrich the flavor of your salad.

- ✔ Tomatoes for salads and sandwiches.

✔ Onions and garlic (in a bowl separate from the others; don't mix your fruit and tomatoes with your garlic and onions).

✔ Avocadoes (if you use them often).

# Cooking with Oils

Part of the Mediterranean lifestyle is using healthy, monounsaturated fats, such as olive oil, in place of butter or other fats. Oils are beneficial for cooking because they allow you to cook food at a higher temperature, and they provide flavor and texture to your foods. The following sections give you the lowdown on cooking with oils to assure you get the healthy benefits.

Although the oils typically associated with the Mediterranean diet are healthier than other oils, they can turn your healthy strategy into an unhealthy one quickly if you aren't careful. As with any fat, you don't want to consume large amounts. Also, oils that are too old or have been stored at the wrong temperature are no good. Taste your oil immediately when you open it so you can see what it tastes like in its freshest form.

## Understanding smoke points

All oils have what's called a *smoke point,* or the temperature at which the fat begins to break down, turning your healthy fat into an unhealthy fat. You want to avoid cooking oils at high temperatures so you don't hit that point of no return. You know when your oil has reached the smoke point because you can actually see smoke and smell a burnt oil or burnt pan odor.

Keep in mind that an oil's smoke point will change depending on how many times you've opened your oil (which brings in oxygen) and how long it's been sitting on the shelf. Don't go higher than medium-high heat when using olive oil; if you see smoke coming off your pan, it's time to start over.

## Distinguishing among types of olive oils

When you start to peruse the oil aisle at the grocery store, you see all sorts of language on the labels like *virgin, extra-virgin,* and *like a virgin* (okay, that last one is in the music aisle). And then you've got *cold-pressed* and *expeller-pressed* to deal with. If you're new to reading these labels, the first thing you need to know about is the manufacturing process.

The hand presses that traditionally pressed olive paste into oil make only a small amount. To increase the output, hot water is added to the presses to get more flow. *Cold-pressed* and *first-pressed* are synonymous labels that indicate that the oil was pressed with little processing in a temperature-controlled environment. *Expeller-pressing* uses the same process as cold-pressing but without the temperature control; it uses heat and friction, but no chemicals or solvents, to create a pure oil with no risk of chemical residues.

Here's a crib sheet of olive oil terminology so that you can become a master at picking out oils:

- ✔ **Extra-virgin olive oil:** All oils produced by the first pressing (the cold pressing) and that contain less than 1 percent acidity, providing rich flavor perfect for drizzling on salads, veggies, or bread.

✔ **Virgin olive oil:** Not as pure as the extra-virgin simply because it uses riper olives, making the acidity higher at 1½ percent. The flavor is still great, but this oil works best as a cooking oil so that you can save the purer-flavored extra-virgin stuff for drizzling.

✔ **Refined olive oil:** A lower-grade olive oil where virgin olive oils with a higher acidity are refined using chemical or physical filters, creating a less-tasty oil with a higher acidity of up to 3 percent. Some places deem this type unfit for human consumption based on flavor.

✔ **Olive oil:** Your basic olive oil is a combination of refined olive oil and virgin olive oil, with a higher quality of flavor than the straight refined olive oil and a 1-percent acidity. This oil works well for basic cooking needs.

✔ **Light olive oil:** The term *light* in this circumstance has nothing to do with calories or fat; rather, it refers to the flavor and color. Light olive oil is made with a fine filtration process and has a very light, almost neutral flavor that won't be so great in your next salad but is a wonderful choice in baking, where you don't want a strong flavor.

✔ **Olive Oyl:** Goes well with spinach.

## Identifying the best oils for different dishes

The world of oils varies greatly in flavor, so you want to have a basic understanding of which oils work best for the different dishes you'll be making in your new Mediterranean lifestyle. You can't go wrong with a basic olive oil or extra-virgin olive oil.

Keep these general tips in mind as you search for oil:

✔ When cooking large recipes, stick with a basic olive oil or extra-virgin olive oil.

✔ When drizzling olive oil on vegetables or dipping your bread, go with a high-quality extra-virgin olive oil.

✔ When you want a little extra punch, try an olive oil flavored with fresh herbs, vinegars, garlic, or lemon juices. Specialty olive oils get pricey, though, so you want to use them lightly.

 To find a good olive oil, visit an olive oil store. The tasting room is set up like a wine tasting. Purchase a good all-purpose olive oil for cooking and one or two specialty olive oils for salads and dipping. You can also purchase decent olive oil at any major grocery store chain or your local farmers' market. If you're intrigued by the specialty oils but can't find them in your area, one great store is the Temecula Olive Oil Company at www.temeculaoliveoil.com.

## Storing oils

Keep your oils in a cool, dark cabinet away from sunlight and heat. You can also store your main cooking oils, such as basic olive oil, in the refrigerator. To avoid storing your oil for too long, buy only a small- to medium-sized glass bottle so that you use it quickly enough.

 If you have a high-quality extra-virgin olive oil, avoid keeping it in the refrigerator; refrigerating increases the risk of condensation. Put the lid on tightly after each use to avoid oxidation, which can turn olive oil rancid. After you open a bottle of oil, store it for up to 6 months. If you're using it frequently, you won't have to worry about it wasting away on your shelf.

# *A Pinch of This and a Pinch of That: Using Herbs and Spices*

People in the Mediterranean use an abundant amount of fresh herbs and spices in their cooking. Besides providing taste, color, and aroma, herbs and spices also add health benefits to your meals.

Do you tend to use a lot of herbs and spices in your cooking, or do you mostly depend on salt and pepper? If you don't use many seasonings, your Mediterranean goal is to cook with more of them, both for the health benefits and to create amazing flavor in your food. This section lets you in on some interesting health benefits simple seasonings provide, how to store the seasonings, and how you can work more of them into your diet.

## *Looking at the health benefits of herbs and spices*

You may have thought that the oregano and basil in your spaghetti sauce just provided a distinct Italian flavor, but those little herbs are plants, which means they have all sorts of health benefits that can make a big impact on your overall health. Simple seasonings such as ginger and oregano contain *phytochemicals,* which are natural health-promoting substances that have been found to protect against conditions such as cancer and heart disease. (Flip to Chapter 2 for more on the powers of phytochemicals.)

Herbs and spices are also loaded with healthy omega-3 fatty acids, which help decrease inflammation in the body. Check out some of the specific health benefits of commonly used herbs and spices:

✔ Basil is shown to have anti-inflammatory effects and may be useful for people with chronic inflammation, such as arthritis or inflammatory bowel disease. Basil also protects against bacteria and is an excellent source of vitamin A, which helps reduce damage to the body from free radicals. (Chapter 2 has more information on vitamin A's benefits.)

✔ Cinnamon helps people better control their blood sugars because it slows digestion and therefore the rise of blood sugar.

✔ Oregano is a nutrient-dense spice containing fiber, iron, manganese, calcium, vitamin C, vitamin A, and omega-3 fatty acids. It's shown to have antibacterial and antioxidant properties.

✔ Parsley is a rich source of the antioxidants vitamin A and vitamin C, providing protection from heart disease and cancer.

✔ Turmeric acts as a powerful anti-inflammatory and antioxidant, helping protect against arthritis, heart disease, and certain cancers.

## Storing fresh and dried herbs

Herbs are delicate, so you want to make sure you store them properly to retain their best taste and their nutrient value. Use these tips for storage:

✔ **Fresh herbs:** Immediately use them. The longer fresh herbs sit around, the more nutrients they lose. Store them in perforated bags in your refrigerator crisper for up to four days.

✔ **Dried herbs and spices:** Use them within a year of purchase. Keep them in airtight containers away from heat and light. You may want to record your date of purchase on the label.

One way to ensure that herbs and seasonings don't sit too long on the shelf is to use them generously in your cooking. If you're running out of dried herbs every six months or so, you're on the right track!

## Livening up food with herbs and spices

With all the health benefits of herbs and spices we note in the preceding section, figuring out a way to increase the herbs and spices in your diet, whether you currently use a moderate amount or none at all, is a great idea. Doing so adds lots of flavor on top of the health perks, so it really is a win-win situation. Here are some suggestions for getting more herbs and spices in your diet:

- ✔ Add ample amounts of herbs to your stews, soups, and chilis. Don't be shy.

- ✔ Use fresh basil leaves in sandwiches, or spread your bread with basil pesto rather than with mayonnaise.

- ✔ Spice up a tuna- or chicken-salad sandwich with some curry, turmeric, and ginger.

- ✔ Let fresh mint, sliced cucumbers, and lemon sit in a pitcher of water for five to ten minutes for a refreshing drink.

- ✔ Mix fresh mint into your next fruit salad.

- ✔ Sprinkle fresh cilantro or basil over black beans and rice for a quick meal.

- ✔ Top off your scrambled eggs with your favorite herb combination.

- ✔ Kick up your lettuce-and-vegetable salads with cilantro and dill.

- ✔ Add fresh dill to fish.

# Chapter 5

# Making Mediterranean-style Main Dishes

## In This Chapter

▶ Exploring quick and tasty breakfast ideas

▶ Staying light with soup, stew, or salad

▶ Preparing pasta masterpieces

▶ Creating pizzas, pitas, and sandwiches

▶ Mastering chicken and seafood dinners

*B*land, boring recipes are something you won't find in Mediterranean cooking. The folks who live on the Mediterranean coast are known for big flavor in all their cooking, and the recipes in this part give you a glimpse.

This chapter includes main dishes for breakfast, lunch, and dinner to demonstrate how you can incorporate more vegetables, healthy fats, and other hallmarks of the Mediterranean diet all day long. Eating right is much easier when the food is this good!

# *Vegetable Omelet*

**Prep time:** 15 min • **Cook time:** 25 min • **Yield:** 4 servings

| Ingredients | Directions |
|---|---|
| 1 tablespoon olive oil<br><br>2 cups thinly sliced fresh fennel bulb<br><br>1 Roma tomato, diced | *1* Preheat the oven to 325 degrees. In a large ovenproof skillet, heat the olive oil over medium-high heat. Add the fennel and sauté for 5 minutes, until soft. |
| ¼ cup pitted green brine-cured olives, chopped<br><br>¼ cup artichoke hearts, marinated in water, rinsed, drained, and chopped | *2* Add in the tomato, olives, and artichoke hearts and sauté for 3 minutes, until softened. |
| 6 eggs<br><br>¼ teaspoon salt<br><br>½ teaspoon pepper | *3* Whisk the eggs in a large bowl and season with the salt and pepper. Pour the whisked eggs into the skillet over the vegetables and stir with a heat-proof spoon for 2 minutes. |
| ½ cup goat cheese, crumbled | *4* Sprinkle the omelet with the cheese and bake for 5 minutes or until the eggs are cooked through and set. |
| 2 tablespoons chopped fresh dill, basil, or parsley | *5* Top with the dill, basil, or parsley. Remove the omelet from the skillet onto a cutting board. Carefully cut the omelet into four wedges, like a pizza, and serve. |

*Per serving:* Calories 152 (From Fat 91); Fat 10g (Saturated 4g); Cholesterol 13mg; Sodium 496mg; Carbohydrate 6g (Dietary Fiber 2g); Protein 11g.

*Vary It!* You can replace the vegetables in this recipe with whatever you have on hand. Some good fits include mushrooms, broccoli, and spinach. Just make sure you sauté them until they're soft before adding your eggs.

# *Zucchini and Goat Cheese Frittata*

**Prep time:** 30 min • **Cook time:** 20 min • **Yield:** 4 servings

| Ingredients | Directions |
|---|---|
| 2 medium zucchinis<br>8 eggs<br>2 tablespoons milk<br>¼ teaspoon salt<br>⅛ teaspoon pepper<br>1 tablespoon olive oil<br>1 clove garlic, crushed<br>2 ounces goat cheese, crumbled | **1** Preheat the oven to 350 degrees. Slice the zucchinis into ¼-inch-thick round slices. In a large bowl, whisk the eggs with the milk, salt, and pepper. |
| | **2** In a heavy, ovenproof skillet (preferably cast iron), heat the olive oil over medium heat. Add the garlic and cook for 30 seconds. Add the zucchini slices and cook for 5 minutes. |
| | **3** Pour the whisked eggs over the zucchini and stir for 1 minute. Top with the cheese and transfer to the oven. Bake for 10 to 12 minutes or until the eggs are set. Remove the pan from the oven and let sit for 3 minutes. |
| | **4** Transfer the frittata to a cutting board, slice into four pie wedges, and serve hot or at room temperature. |

*Per serving:* Calories 134 (From Fat 72); Fat 8g (Saturated 3g); Cholesterol 11mg; Sodium 324mg; Carbohydrate 4g (Dietary Fiber 1g); Protein 12g.

*Vary It!* You can use yellow squash in place of the zucchini.

# *Dilled Eggs*

**Prep time:** 10 min • **Cook time:** 5 min • **Yield:** 4 servings

| *Ingredients* | *Directions* |
|---|---|
| **1 tablespoon olive oil** <br><br> **¼ cup onion, minced** <br><br> **8 eggs** <br><br> **2 tablespoons fresh dill** <br><br> **2 ounces feta, crumbled** <br><br> **Salt and pepper to taste** | *1* In a large nonstick skillet, heat the olive oil over medium heat. Add in the onion and cook for 3 minutes, until softened. Crack the eggs into a medium bowl and then pour them into the pan. <br><br> *2* Whisk the eggs in the pan, breaking each yolk. Stir the eggs every 30 seconds until they set and are firm. <br><br> *3* Add in the dill and cheese. Season with salt and pepper to taste and serve. |

*Per serving:* Calories 103 (From Fat 59); Fat 7g (Saturated 3g); Cholesterol 13mg; Sodium 268mg; Carbohydrate 2g (Dietary Fiber 0g); Protein 9g.

*Vary It!* You can replace the feta with goat cheese.

# Lentil Soup with Tomatoes and Spinach

**Prep time:** 8 min • **Cook time:** 45 min • **Yield:** 8 servings

| Ingredients | Directions |
|---|---|
| 1 tablespoon olive oil | *1* Heat the olive oil in a large stock pot over medium heat. After 1 minute, add the onions, carrot, and celery and cook until the onions are translucent, about 6 to 7 minutes. |
| 1 cup chopped onion | |
| ½ cup carrot, diced small | |
| ½ cup celery, diced small | |
| 1½ teaspoon salt | *2* Add the salt, lentils, tomatoes, broth, coriander, cumin, and bay leaf and stir to combine. Increase the heat to high and bring just to a boil. |
| 1 pound orange or brown lentils | |
| One 14.5-ounce can unsalted chopped tomatoes | |
| 8 cups chicken or vegetable broth | *3* Reduce the heat to low, cover, and cook at a low simmer until the lentils are tender, about 35 to 40 minutes. Add the spinach in during the last 15 minutes or simply add to each bowl for serving. Season with salt and pepper to taste and serve immediately. |
| ½ teaspoon ground coriander | |
| ½ teaspoon ground cumin | |
| 1 bay leaf | |
| 5 ounces baby spinach leaves | |
| Salt and pepper to taste | |

*Per serving: Calories 285 (From Fat 35); Fat 4g (Saturated 1g); Cholesterol 0mg; Sodium 959mg; Carbohydrate 42g (Dietary Fiber 19g); Protein 21g.*

*Tip:* If you want to use a slow cooker, combine all the ingredients except the spinach in the slow cooker and cook for 6 hours on low. Add the spinach during the last 15 minutes of cooking or to each bowl for serving.

# Chicken Stew with Chickpeas and Plum Tomatoes

**Prep time:** 12 min • **Cook time:** 1 hr, 15 min • **Yield:** 6 servings

| Ingredients | Directions |
|---|---|
| 2 tablespoons olive oil<br>4 skinless chicken thighs<br>1 small onion, chopped<br>1 celery stalk, chopped<br>½ teaspoon cinnamon<br>¼ teaspoon ginger<br>1 teaspoon turmeric<br>1 teaspoon pepper<br>½ teaspoon salt<br>One 14.5-ounce can chickpeas, drained | *1* In a large stock pot, heat the olive oil over medium-high heat. Add the chicken thighs and cook for 3 minutes on each side. Add the onion, celery, spices, and chickpeas and cook for 3 minutes to heat the spices. |
| One 28-ounce can whole plum tomatoes, with juice<br>6 cups low-sodium chicken stock<br>¼ cup red lentils<br>½ cup long-grain rice | *2* Pour in the tomatoes (with their juice), stock, lentils, and rice. Bring the mixture to a boil over medium-high heat, cover, reduce the heat to low, and simmer for 1 hour and 15 minutes. |
| ¼ cup lemon juice<br>½ cup cilantro, chopped | *3* Stir in the lemon juice and divide the stew into six bowls. Garnish each bowl with 2 tablespoons of chopped cilantro and serve. |

*Per serving: Calories 346 (From Fat 82); Fat 9g (Saturated 2g); Cholesterol 38mg; Sodium 721mg; Carbohydrate 47g (Dietary Fiber 6g); Protein 22g.*

# Char-Grilled Chicken with Feta over Mixed Greens

**Prep time:** 40 min, plus marinating time • **Cook time:** 20 min • **Yield:** 4 servings

| Ingredients | Directions |
|---|---|
| Four 4- to 6-ounce boneless, skinless chicken breasts | *1*   Place the chicken breasts in a 9-x-11-inch glass baking dish. |
| ½ cup red wine vinegar | *2*   In a small bowl, whisk together the vinegar, olive oil, garlic, mustard, oregano, fennel seed, coriander, and honey. Pour 1 cup of the dressing over the chicken and coat each breast. Marinate the chicken in the refrigerator for 30 minutes to 4 hours. Discard this portion of the dressing. |
| 1 cup olive oil | |
| 2 cloves garlic, chopped | |
| 2 teaspoons yellow mustard | |
| 1 teaspoon dried oregano | *3*   Divide the mixed greens among four plates. Halve each tomato and cut it into ½-inch wedges. Divide the tomatoes, olives, and feta evenly among the plates. |
| ¼ teaspoon fennel seed | |
| ¼ teaspoon coriander | *4*   Remove the chicken from the refrigerator and discard the marinade. Heat a grill or grill pan to medium-high heat. Grill the chicken for 10 minutes on each side or until the internal temperature reaches 165 degrees. |
| 2 teaspoons honey | |
| 8 cups mixed salad greens | |
| 2 Roma tomatoes | *5*   Allow the chicken to rest on a cutting board for 5 minutes prior to slicing. Slice each chicken breast on an angle in ½-inch-thick slices. Fan one breast over each salad. |
| 16 black olives | |
| 4 ounces feta, crumbled | |
| | *6*   Drizzle 1 to 2 tablespoons of the remaining dressing over each salad and serve. |

*Per serving:* Calories 290 (From Fat 92); Fat 10g (Saturated 4g); Cholesterol 126mg; Sodium 576mg; Carbohydrate 7g (Dietary Fiber 1g); Protein 41g.

# Grilled Salmon with Caramelized Onions over Mixed Greens

**Prep time:** 15 min, plus marinating time • **Cook time:** 40 min • **Yield:** 4 servings

| Ingredients | Directions |
|---|---|
| 1 tablespoon plus ¼ cup olive oil | **1** In a heavy skillet, heat 1 tablespoon of the olive oil and 1 tablespoon of butter over medium-high heat. Add the onions and sauté over medium-high heat until slightly soft and caramelized, being careful not to fully brown, for 3 minutes, tossing with tongs to separate pieces and evenly coat with oil mixture. |
| 1 tablespoon butter | |
| 2 large sweet or yellow onions, sliced thinly | |
| 2 tablespoons fresh dill, chopped | **2** Reduce the heat to medium-low and continue sautéing uncovered for 20 to 25 minutes or until golden. |
| 3 cloves garlic, minced | **3** Mix the dill, garlic, lemon zest and juice, remaining olive oil, and melted butter and season with the sea salt to taste. Place all but ¼ cup of the dressing into another bowl and use the ¼ cup to brush both sides of the salmon; marinate for 10 minutes. Discard this portion of the dressing. |
| Zest and juice of 1 lemon | |
| 1 tablespoon butter, melted | |
| ¼ teaspoon sea salt, or to taste | **4** Heat a grill or grill pan to medium-high heat. Grill the salmon on each side for 4 minutes or until it achieves the desired doneness. |
| 1 pound salmon fillet | |
| 4 cups romaine lettuce | **5** In a large mixing bowl, lightly toss the greens with the reserved dressing and plate on four dinner plates. |
| 4 cups red leaf lettuce | **6** Divide the caramelized onions evenly among the four plates. Cut the salmon into four equal pieces and plate them over the onions; sprinkle with the chopped walnuts and serve hot. |
| ¼ cup walnuts or almonds, chopped | |

*Per serving:* Calories 322 (From Fat 161); Fat 18g (Saturated 5g); Cholesterol 74mg; Sodium 290mg; Carbohydrate 15g (Dietary Fiber 3g); Protein 27g.

# *Puttanesca*

**Prep time:** 8 min • **Cook time:** 23 min • **Yield:** 6 servings

| Ingredients | Directions |
|---|---|
| **One 12-ounce box penne** | *1*   Bring 4 quarts of water to a boil. Cook the pasta according to the package directions (8 to 12 minutes). Drain the pasta, reserving 1 cup of pasta water. |
| **½ cup extra-virgin olive oil** | |
| **3 cloves garlic, chopped** | *2*   Meanwhile, heat the olive oil in a saucepan over medium heat. Add the garlic and red pepper flakes and cook for 30 seconds. Stir in the tomatoes, oregano, olives, capers, and tomato paste; increase the heat to medium-high and cook for 10 minutes. |
| **1 teaspoon red pepper flakes** | |
| **One 28-ounce can Italian plum tomatoes** | |
| **1½ teaspoons dried oregano** | *3*   Add the cooked pasta to the sauce and toss. If the sauce is too thick, add the reserved pasta water ¼ cup at a time until you reach the desired consistency. |
| **½ cup pitted kalamata olives, chopped** | |
| **3 tablespoons capers, drained and rinsed** | |
| **2 tablespoons tomato paste** | *4*   Top with chopped parsley and grated Parmesan and serve. |
| **¼ cup fresh Italian parsley, chopped** | |
| **¼ cup finely grated Parmesan cheese** | |

*Per serving: Calories 428 (From Fat 192); Fat 21g (Saturated 4g); Cholesterol 4mg; Sodium 528mg; Carbohydrate 50g (Dietary Fiber 4g); Protein 11g.*

# Baked Eggplant Parmesan with Linguini

**Prep time:** 30 min • **Cook time:** 15 min • **Yield:** 8 servings

| Ingredients | Directions |
|---|---|
| **1 cup flour** <br> **1 teaspoon salt** <br> **1 teaspoon pepper** <br> **2 eggs** <br> **¼ cup water** <br> **1 teaspoon dried oregano** <br> **3 cups panko breadcrumbs** <br> **2 medium eggplants** <br> **½ of a lemon** <br> **¼ cup olive oil** <br> **4 ounces fresh mozzarella** <br> **1 pound linguini** <br> **4 cups roasted red pepper sauce or Marinara** | *1* Preheat the oven to 400 degrees. Combine the flour, salt, and pepper in a medium bowl. Whisk together the eggs and water in another medium bowl, and combine the panko and oregano in a third. <br><br> *2* Remove the stem and bottom of the eggplant and cut ½-inch thick slices lengthwise. Rub the cut portion of the eggplant with the lemon wedge to stop browning. <br><br> *3* Dip the eggplant in the flour and dust off the excess; dip the floured eggplant into the egg mixture and then the panko. Set aside on a large plate and repeat with the remaining eggplant. <br><br> *4* Meanwhile, heat 1 tablespoon of the olive oil in a heavy cast-iron Dutch oven or skillet on medium-high heat. Working in batches, brown the breaded eggplants for about 3 minutes on each side, being careful not to crowd the pan. <br><br> *5* Transfer to a baking sheet. Repeat with the remaining eggplant, using 1 tablespoon of olive oil for each batch. Top each eggplant with a thin slice of fresh mozzarella and bake for 15 minutes. <br><br> *6* Bring 3 quarts of water to a boil. Cook the linguini according to the package instructions and drain. Divide the linguini evenly on 8 serving plates, cover with ½ cup of heated sauce and top with the eggplant Parmesan. Serve. |

*Per serving:* Calories 550 (From Fat 140); Fat 16g (Saturated 4g); Cholesterol 12mg; Sodium 1350mg; Carbohydrate 84g (Dietary Fiber 11g); Protein 18g.

# *Pizza Dough*

**Prep time:** 25 min • **Yield:** 1 pizza, 10 servings

| Ingredients | Directions |
|---|---|
| **One ¼-ounce package active dry yeast** | *1* Combine the yeast, honey, and warm water in a large mixer or food processor with a dough attachment. Let the mixture rest for 5 minutes to be sure that the yeast is alive (look for bubbles on the surface). |
| **2 teaspoons honey** | |
| **1¼ cups warm water (about 110 to 120 degrees)** | |
| **2 tablespoons olive oil** | *2* Add the olive oil and salt and blend for 30 seconds. Begin to slowly add the flour, about ½ cup at a time, mixing for 2 minutes between additions. |
| **1 teaspoon sea salt** | |
| **3 cups flour** | |
| | *3* Allow the mixture to knead in the mixer for 10 minutes, sprinkling with flour if needed to keep the dough from sticking to the bowl, until elastic and smooth. |
| | *4* Remove the dough from the bowl and allow it to rest for 15 minutes under a warm, moist towel. See the following pizza recipe for baking instructions. |

*Per serving: Calories 167 (From Fat 28); Fat 3g (Saturated 0g); Cholesterol 0mg; Sodium 234mg; Carbohydrate 30g (Dietary Fiber 1g); Protein 4g.*

*Note:* You can freeze this pizza dough for 1 month. Form the dough into a ball and cover it with plastic wrap before placing it into a freezer-safe container.

# *Sausage and Pepper Pizza*

**Prep time:** 15 min • **Cook time:** 25 min • **Yield:** 10 servings

| *Ingredients* | *Directions* |
|---|---|
| 1 batch Pizza Dough<br><br>¼ cup flour as needed for rolling<br><br>1 tablespoon olive oil<br><br>1 onion, thinly sliced<br><br>1 green bell pepper, julienned<br><br>½ teaspoon sea salt<br><br>1 cup pizza sauce<br><br>½ pound Italian sausage, casing removed<br><br>½ pound cremini mushrooms, quartered<br><br>8 ounces fontina cheese, grated<br><br>½ teaspoon dried oregano | *1* Preheat the oven to 450 degrees. Roll out the pizza dough about ½-inch thick into your desired shape and place it onto a parchment paper-lined baking sheet.<br><br>*2* Heat the olive oil in a nonstick skillet over medium-high heat. Add the onions and peppers and cook for 5 minutes. Remove from the heat and season with sea salt.<br><br>*3* Spread the pizza sauce onto the pizza dough and top with the pepper and onion mixture. Form ½-inch balls with the sausage and add them and the mushrooms to the pizza. Top the pizza with the cheese and sprinkle with the dried oregano.<br><br>*4* Bake the pizza for 15 to 20 minutes or until the cheese is browned. Remove the pizza from the oven and let it cool for 5 minutes before serving. |

*Per serving:* Calories 389 (From Fat 171); Fat 19g (Saturated 7g); Cholesterol 44mg; Sodium 748mg; Carbohydrate 39g (Dietary Fiber 2g); Protein 15g.

*Note:* Be sure to form the sausage into small (½-inch) balls to ensure even and complete cooking time. Test your sausage prior to serving to make sure it's cooked through. If it's not, place the pizza back in the oven and continue cooking until the sausage is no longer pink.

# Roasted Vegetables with Feta Cheese Pita

**Prep time:** 15 min • **Cook time:** 5 min • **Yield:** 4 servings

| Ingredients | Directions |
|---|---|
| **1 red bell pepper, cut into 1-inch pieces** | *1* In a broiler-safe baking dish, toss together the peppers, tomatoes, and chickpeas. Drizzle with the olive oil and broil 5 to 7 inches from the heating element for 5 to 8 minutes or until slightly blackened. |
| **1 yellow bell pepper, cut into 1-inch pieces** | |
| **1 green bell pepper, cut into 1-inch pieces** | |
| **1 large tomato, cut into ½-inch wedges** | *2* Meanwhile, in a large bowl, combine the lemon juice, garlic, parsley, cumin, and salt. After the veggies are broiled, immediately toss them in the vinaigrette. |
| **One 14.5-ounce can chickpeas, drained and rinsed** | |
| **¼ cup olive oil** | |
| **Juice of 1 lemon** | *3* Heat the pitas or flatbreads on a hot griddle or in a cast-iron skillet for 3 to 5 minutes or until hot. Fill each sandwich with vegetables and top with 2 tablespoons of feta. Serve immediately. |
| **2 cloves garlic, minced** | |
| **½ cup parsley, chopped** | |
| **¼ teaspoon ground cumin** | |
| **½ teaspoon salt** | |
| **4 pita pockets or flatbreads** | |
| **½ cup feta cheese, crumbled** | |

*Per serving: Calories 397 (From Fat 175); Fat 19g (Saturated 5g); Cholesterol 17mg; Sodium 841mg; Carbohydrate 46g (Dietary Fiber 7g); Protein 12g.*

# Oven-Fried Fish Sandwich with Fresh Spring Mix

**Prep time:** 15 min • **Cook time:** 20 min • **Yield:** 6 servings

| Ingredients | Directions |
|---|---|
| ½ cup flour | **1** Preheat the oven to 425 degrees. |
| ½ teaspoon garlic powder | |
| ¼ teaspoon paprika | **2** In a medium bowl, combine the flour, garlic powder, paprika, and salt. In another bowl, combine the egg and Greek yogurt; place the bread crumbs in a third bowl. |
| ⅛ teaspoon salt | |
| 1 egg | |
| ½ cup Greek yogurt | |
| 1 cup panko breadcrumbs | **3** Dredge the fish in the flour mixture and shake off any excess. Dip the floured fish into the yogurt mixture and then coat it with the breadcrumbs. Place the breaded fish onto a baking sheet. |
| Four 6-ounce fillets flounder or other white fish | |
| ¼ cup grated Parmesan cheese | **4** Bake the fish for 20 minutes or until golden. Immediately upon removing from the oven, top each fillet with 1 tablespoon of Parmesan cheese. |
| 1 French bread baguette | |
| 2 cups spring mix lettuce | **5** Cut the baguette in half lengthwise and top it with the cooked fish. In a medium bowl, toss the greens with the lemon juice and olive oil to coat; season to taste with salt and pepper. |
| Juice of 1 lemon | |
| 2 tablespoons extra-virgin olive oil | |
| Salt and pepper to taste | **6** Place the greens over the fish, cut the sandwich into 4 servings, and serve. |

*Per serving:* Calories 424 (From Fat 82); Fat 9g (Saturated 2g); Cholesterol 58mg; Sodium 706mg; Carbohydrate 49g (Dietary Fiber 2g); Protein 35g.

# Sautéed Chicken Breasts in Red Wine Tomato Sauce

**Prep time:** 10 min • **Cook time:** 45 min • **Yield:** 4 servings

| *Ingredients* | *Directions* |
|---|---|
| **Four 4-ounce bone-in, skin-on chicken breasts** | *1* Preheat the oven to 350 degrees. Rub the chicken with 2 tablespoons oil and season with the salt and pepper. |
| **2 tablespoons plus 2 tablespoons olive oil** | |
| **¼ teaspoon salt** | |
| **½ teaspoon pepper** | *2* Heat the remaining olive oil in a heavy ovenproof (preferably cast-iron) Dutch oven over medium-high heat. Brown the chicken for 4 minutes on each side and remove it from the pan and set aside. |
| **1 tablespoon fennel seeds** | |
| **2 celery stalks, chopped** | |
| **½ of a medium onion, chopped** | |
| **4 cloves garlic, sliced** | *3* Add the fennel seeds, celery, onion, and garlic and cook for 3 minutes, stirring frequently. Add the red pepper flakes and olives, cook for 1 minute, and return the chicken to the pan. Add the tomatoes and stir in the wine. |
| **1 teaspoon red pepper flakes** | |
| **¼ cup black kalamata olives, pitted** | |
| **One 14.8-ounce can tomatoes, chopped** | |
| **1 cup spicy red wine, such as a red Zinfandel** | |
| **2 tablespoons parsley, chopped** | *4* Bake for 30 minutes. Top the chicken with the parsley and mint and serve. |
| **2 tablespoons mint, chopped** | |

*Per serving: Calories 343 (From Fat 175); Fat 19g (Saturated 3g); Cholesterol 50mg; Sodium 649mg; Carbohydrate 12g (Dietary Fiber 3g); Protein 20g.*

# Grilled Yogurt Chicken with Mint

**Prep time:** 30 min, plus marinating time • **Cook time:** 10 min • **Yield:** 6 servings

| Ingredients | Directions |
|---|---|
| **One 5-pound whole chicken, butterflied** | **1** Place the butterflied chicken into a glass baking pan. Combine the remaining ingredients and pour the mixture over the chicken to coat both sides. Marinate the chicken in the refrigerator for 4 to 8 hours. |
| **1 cup plain Greek yogurt** | |
| **2 tablespoons extra-virgin olive oil** | |
| **4 cloves garlic, minced** | **2** Heat the grill over medium heat. Shake off any excess marinade, place the chicken on the grill skin side down, and cook for 15 minutes on each side. Flip the chicken again and finish cooking with the skin side down until the thickest part of the chicken reads 165 degrees. |
| **1 whole lemon, chopped** | |
| **⅓ cup fresh mint, chopped** | |
| **2 teaspoons ground cumin** | |
| **½ teaspoon cayenne pepper** | **3** Remove the chicken from the grill and cover with foil; allow the chicken to rest for 15 minutes before serving. Slice the chicken and serve 2 to 3 ounces per serving. |
| **1 teaspoon coarse salt** | |

***Per serving:*** *Calories 261 (From Fat 83); Fat 9g (Saturated 2g); Cholesterol 113mg; Sodium 536mg; Carbohydrate 4g (Dietary Fiber 1g); Protein 40g.*

# Grilled Tuna with Braised Fennel

**Prep time:** 8 min • **Cook time:** 16 min • **Yield:** 4 servings

| Ingredients | Directions |
|---|---|
| ¼ cup plus 1 tablespoon olive oil | **1** Preheat the grill over medium-high heat. |
| 2 fennel bulbs, sliced ¼-inch thick | |
| 1 onion, sliced in ¼-inch slices | **2** In a heavy skillet, heat ¼ cup of the olive oil over medium heat. Add the fennel, onions, and garlic and sauté for 8 minutes, stirring frequently. Add the olives and capers and cook over low heat for 5 minutes. |
| 3 cloves garlic, chopped | |
| ¼ cup kalamata olives, pitted and chopped | **3** Brush the fish with the remaining olive oil and season lightly with salt and pepper. Grill the fish for 3 minutes on each side or until slightly rare in the center. |
| ¼ cup capers, drained and rinsed | |
| Four 6-ounce yellowtail tuna fillets | |
| ¼ cup parsley, chopped | **4** Add the parsley and lemon juice to the fennel mixture, season with salt, stir, and serve over the fish. |
| Juice of 2 lemons | |
| Salt and pepper to taste | |

***Per serving:*** *Calories 345 (From Fat 172); Fat 19g (Saturated 3g); Cholesterol 51mg; Sodium 439mg; Carbohydrate 16g (Dietary Fiber 5g); Protein 29g.*

# Sautéed Shrimp with White Wine and Feta

**Prep time:** 5 min  •  **Cook time:** 12 min  •  **Yield:** 6 servings

| Ingredients | Directions |
|---|---|
| 1 tablespoon olive oil | **1**  Heat the olive oil in a large nonstick skillet over medium heat. Add the red pepper flakes and onion and sauté for 3 minutes. Add the garlic and cook for 3 minutes. |
| ½ teaspoon red pepper flakes | |
| ½ of a medium onion, cut into ¼-inch slices | |
| 6 cloves garlic, sliced | **2**  Season the shrimp with salt and pepper; add them to the skillet and sauté for 2 minutes per side. Add the wine and parsley and cook for 1 minute or until the shrimp is cooked. Crumble the feta over the top and serve. |
| 2 pounds shrimp, peeled and deveined | |
| Salt and pepper to taste | |
| ½ cup white wine | |
| ¼ cup parsley, chopped | |
| ¼ cup feta, crumbled | |

*Per serving:* Calories 222 (From Fat 56); Fat 6g (Saturated 2g); Cholesterol 235mg; Sodium 297mg; Carbohydrate 4g (Dietary Fiber 0g); Protein 32g.

# Chapter 6

# Stepping Up the Flavor with Side Dishes

. . . . . . . . . . . . . . . . . . . . . .

*In This Chapter*

▶ Keeping it cool with yogurt sauce and salads

▶ Getting your veggies on the side

▶ Trying your hand at whole grains

▶ Inviting beans and lentils onto your plate

. . . . . . . . . . . . . . . . . . . . . .

*Recipes in This Chapter*

↻ Cucumber Yogurt Sauce
↻ Tomato, Cucumber, and Basil Salad
↻ Pomegranate Salad
↻ Roasted Broccoli and Tomatoes
↻ Sautéed Eggplant with Tomatoes and Black Olives
↻ Garlic and Lemon Roasted Potatoes
↻ Curry-Roasted Cauliflower
↻ Grilled Fennel
▶ Rice-Stuffed Tomatoes
▶ Golden Pilaf
↻ Bulgur Salad with White Beans and Spinach
↻ Spinach and Lentils with Feta
↻ Beet and Kidney Bean Salad
↻ Savory Fava Beans with Warm Pita Bread
↻ Falafel

🍴🧅🍲🌶🖐🌿

*T*ired of serving white rice, mashed potatoes, and plain steamed vegetables with your meals? You've come to the right chapter. You can add some truly flavorful and interesting side dishes to your table with the Mediterranean diet.

You have endless possibilities when it comes to Mediterranean-style side dishes. In this chapter, we hope to whet your appetite by showing a delicious sampling of what you can do with key Mediterranean diet ingredients such as vegetables, whole grains, legumes, herbs, and spices. Let these ideas inspire you to seek out even more recipes so your main dishes are never bored with their companions!

# *Cucumber Yogurt Sauce*

**Prep time:** 5 min • **Yield:** 12 servings

| *Ingredients* | *Directions* |
| --- | --- |
| **2 cups Greek yogurt** <br><br> **1 cucumber, peeled and seeded** <br><br> **Zest and juice of 1 lemon** <br><br> **¼ cup mint, minced** <br><br> **2 cloves garlic, minced** | *1* Place yogurt into a bowl. Grate the cucumber into the yogurt and stir. Season the yogurt mixture with the remaining ingredients. Store in the refrigerator until ready to serve. |

*Per serving: Calories 24 (From Fat 0); Fat 0g (Saturated 0g); Cholesterol 0mg; Sodium 18mg; Carbohydrate 2g (Dietary Fiber 0g); Protein 4g.*

*Tip:* This sauce makes a great addition to any grilled meat or kabobs.

*Note:* Store in the refrigerator for up to a week.

# Tomato, Cucumber, and Basil Salad

**Prep time:** 12 min • **Yield:** 8 servings

| Ingredients | Directions |
|---|---|
| **8 Roma tomatoes** | *1* Slice each tomato into 6 wedges. Cut off both ends of the cucumber and slice it lengthwise down the middle. With a spoon, scrape out the seeds. Slice the cucumber into half moons about ¼-inch thick. |
| **1 large cucumber** | |
| **¼ cup red onion, cut into ⅛-inch slices and then halved** | |
| **¼ cup fresh basil leaves, cut into thin strips** | *2* In a large serving bowl, toss together everything but the salt and pepper. Season with salt and pepper and serve. |
| **2 tablespoons olive oil** | |
| **3 tablespoons balsamic vinegar** | |
| **¼ cup feta cheese** | |
| **Salt and pepper to taste** | |

*Per serving: Calories 65 (From Fat 41); Fat 5g (Saturated 1g); Cholesterol 4mg; Sodium 58mg; Carbohydrate 5g (Dietary Fiber 1g); Protein 2g.*

# Pomegranate Salad

**Prep time:** 8 min • **Cook time:** 7 min • **Yield:** 4 servings

| Ingredients | Directions |
|---|---|
| 2 tablespoons plus 2 tablespoons olive oil<br><br>8 ounces chilled halloumi cheese, cut into ¼-inch-thick slices | *1* In a large, heavy cast-iron or nonstick skillet, heat 2 tablespoons of the oil over medium-high heat. Add the cheese, being careful not to crowd the pan, and lower the temperature to medium-low. |
| 6 cups baby arugula leaves or spinach<br><br>1 cup fresh mint leaves, sliced into long, thin strips | *2* Cook the cheese for 2 minutes on each side or until a golden brown crust is achieved. Place the cooked cheese on paper towels to drain; remove the excess oil from the pan and reserve for the salad. |
| ½ cup pistachios<br><br>½ cup pomegranate seeds | *3* In a serving bowl, toss together the arugula, mint, pistachios, and pomegranate seeds. |
| ¼ cup bottled pomegranate juice<br><br>1 tablespoon lemon juice<br><br>Salt and pepper to taste | *4* In a small saucepan, heat the pomegranate juice over medium heat until it reduces by half, about 3 minutes. Remove from the heat, add the remaining olive oil and the lemon juice, and season with salt and pepper to taste. |
| | *5* Toss the salad mixture with ¼ cup of the dressing. Arrange the cheese slices on top of the salad, drizzle with the remainder of the dressing, and serve. |

***Per serving:*** *Calories 419 (From Fat 307); Fat 34g (Saturated 10g); Cholesterol 45mg; Sodium 418mg; Carbohydrate 14g (Dietary Fiber 4g); Protein 18g.*

*Note:* Halloumi cheese is a popular cheese used in Greece and found in specialty stores. You can also buy it online. If you can't find it, buy slices of mozzarella cheese; brush them with egg whites and dust with bread crumbs prior to cooking so they don't melt.

# *Roasted Broccoli and Tomatoes*

**Prep time:** 8 min • **Cook time:** 15 min • **Yield:** 4 servings

| Ingredients | Directions |
|---|---|
| **1 pound broccoli** | *1* Preheat the oven to 450 degrees. Cut off the broccoli florets with a 1-inch stem on each crown. Peel the remaining stalk with a vegetable peeler and cut into 1-inch-long pieces. |
| **2 cups Roma or cherry tomatoes** | |
| **1 tablespoon olive oil** | |
| **2 tablespoons balsamic vinegar** | *2* Place the broccoli and ¼ cup of water into a microwave-safe bowl; microwave the broccoli for 3 minutes to soften. Drain and pat dry. |
| **¼ teaspoon sugar or honey** | |
| **1 teaspoon dried oregano** | *3* Quarter the tomatoes and toss with the broccoli. Drizzle the veggies with olive oil, toss, and spread onto a baking sheet. Roast for 12 to 15 minutes or until the broccoli begins to lightly brown. |
| **1 clove garlic, minced** | |
| **Salt to taste** | |
| | *4* Meanwhile, combine the balsamic vinegar, sugar, oregano, and garlic. As soon as the vegetables come out of the oven, place them in a serving bowl and drizzle with the balsamic dressing. Toss and serve. |

***Per serving:*** *Calories 90 (From Fat 35); Fat 4g (Saturated 1g); Cholesterol 0mg; Sodium 43mg; Carbohydrate 12g (Dietary Fiber 4g); Protein 4g.*

# Sautéed Eggplant with Tomatoes and Black Olives

**Prep time:** 10 min • **Cook time:** 30 min • **Yield:** 6 servings

| Ingredients | Directions |
|---|---|
| 2 tablespoons olive oil<br><br>3 cloves garlic, chopped | *1* In a heavy skillet, heat the olive oil over medium heat. Add the garlic, eggplant, and oregano and sauté for 10 minutes. |
| 1 large eggplant, unpeeled, cut into ½-inch cubes<br><br>1 tablespoon dried oregano<br><br>One 28-ounce can no-salt-added diced tomatoes | *2* Add the tomatoes, olives, tomato paste, and red wine vinegar and reduce the heat to medium-low. Cover and cook until the eggplant softens, stirring often, about 15 minutes. If needed, occasionally add 1 tablespoon of water to the pan to help the eggplant soften and cook. |
| ¼ cup kalamata or black olives<br><br>¼ cup tomato paste<br><br>2 tablespoons red wine vinegar<br><br>1 to 3 tablespoons water<br><br>1 cup fresh basil, sliced thinly<br><br>Salt and pepper to taste<br><br>¼ cup ricotta cheese | *3* Stir in the basil and simmer for 3 to 5 minutes. Season with salt and pepper to taste. Place into a serving dish, dollop with spoonfuls of the ricotta, and serve. |

*Per serving:* Calories 118 (From Fat 61); Fat 7g (Saturated 2g); Cholesterol 5mg; Sodium 164mg; Carbohydrate 13g (Dietary Fiber 5g); Protein 4g.

# *Garlic and Lemon Roasted Potatoes*

**Prep time:** 6 min • **Cook time:** 35 min • **Yield:** 6 servings

| Ingredients | Directions |
|---|---|
| 1½ pounds fingerling or new potatoes<br><br>3 tablespoons olive oil<br><br>3 cloves garlic, minced<br><br>½ teaspoon dried oregano<br><br>½ teaspoon pepper<br><br>Zest of 1 lemon (about 1 tablespoon)<br><br>¼ teaspoon sea salt | *1* Preheat the oven to 425 degrees. Slice the potatoes in half (for fingerling) or quarters (for new) and place them on a baking sheet or roasting pan.<br><br>*2* Drizzle the potatoes with the olive oil, garlic, and oregano and toss to coat. Bake the potatoes for 20 minutes; gently stir. Continue cooking for an additional 15 minutes or until golden brown. Remove from the oven and place into a serving bowl.<br><br>*3* Toss the warm potatoes with the pepper, zest, and sea salt to serve. |

*Per serving: Calories 139 (From Fat 62); Fat 7g (Saturated 1g); Cholesterol 0mg; Sodium 104mg; Carbohydrate 18g (Dietary Fiber 2g); Protein 2g.*

# Curry-Roasted Cauliflower

**Prep time:** 6 min • **Cook time:** 35 min • **Yield:** 6 servings

| Ingredients | Directions |
|---|---|
| 1 head cauliflower | *1* Preheat the oven to 425 degrees. |
| ¼ cup olive oil | |
| ½ cup red wine vinegar | *2* Cut the cauliflower (including the stalk and leaves) into bite-sized pieces and place in a medium bowl. |
| 1 teaspoon ground coriander | |
| 1 teaspoon ground cumin | *3* In a small bowl, whisk the remaining ingredients. Pour over the cauliflower and toss to coat. |
| 1 tablespoon curry powder | |
| 1 tablespoon paprika | *4* Pour the cauliflower and sauce onto a baking sheet and bake for 35 minutes, stirring every 5 minutes. Serve. |
| 1 teaspoon salt | |

*Per serving:* Calories 118 (From Fat 85); Fat 9g (Saturated 1g); Cholesterol 0mg; Sodium 431mg; Carbohydrate 7g (Dietary Fiber 3g); Protein 3g.

# *Grilled Fennel*

**Prep time:** 5 min • **Cook time:** 8 min • **Yield:** 4 servings

| Ingredients | Directions |
|---|---|
| **2 fennel bulbs**<br><br>**1 tablespoon plus 1 tablespoon olive oil**<br><br>**⅛ teaspoon salt**<br><br>**⅛ teaspoon red pepper flakes**<br><br>**1 orange**<br><br>**¼ cup raw almonds, chopped** | *1* Heat a grill over medium-high heat. Cut the fennel bulbs in half, drizzle them with 1 tablespoon of the olive oil, and season with the salt and red pepper flakes. Grill the fennel for 4 to 6 minutes on each side. |
| | *2* Using a sharp knife, cut the skin away from the orange, removing the white outer portion. Cut the orange in half, break it into segments. |
| | *3* Toast the almonds in a skillet over medium heat for 3 to 4 minutes, stirring or tossing constantly to avoid burning. Sprinkle the almonds over the orange slices. |
| | *4* Thinly slice the fennel and toss it with the orange slices and almonds. Drizzle with the remaining olive oil and serve. |

*Per serving:* *Calories 169 (From Fat 103); Fat 11g (Saturated 1g); Cholesterol 0mg; Sodium 235mg; Carbohydrate 16g (Dietary Fiber 6g); Protein 4g.*

# Rice-Stuffed Tomatoes

**Prep time:** 15 min • **Cook time:** 1 hr • **Yield:** 6 servings

| *Ingredients* | *Directions* |
|---|---|
| **6 medium tomatoes** <br> **1 cup white rice** <br> **1½ cups chicken stock** <br> **¼ cup plus 1 cup white wine** <br> **1 bay leaf** <br> **1 teaspoon olive oil** <br> **⅓ cup plus 6 teaspoons grated Parmesan cheese** <br> **¼ cup green onions, chopped** <br> **¼ cup fresh basil leaves, chopped** | *1* Cut ½-inch caps off the tops of the tomatoes and set aside. Carefully scoop out the tomato pulp and put it into a medium saucepan. Put the hollowed tomatoes upright into an 8-x-8-inch baking dish. |
| | *2* Heat the saucepan over medium high heat, add the rice to the tomato pulp, and cook for 1 minute. Add the stock, ¼ cup of the wine, the bay leaf, and the olive oil and bring to a boil. |
| | *3* Reduce the heat to a simmer and cover for 20 to 25 minutes or until the liquid is absorbed. Discard the bay leaf. Remove the pot from the heat and allow the rice mixture to cool for 10 minutes. |
| | *4* Preheat the oven to 350 degrees. Stir in ⅓ cup of the Parmesan, the green onions, and basil to the cooled rice. Fill the tomatoes with rice mixture. |
| | *5* Top each tomato with 1 teaspoon of Parmesan cheese. Place the top onto each tomato and lightly cover the pan with foil. |
| | *6* Bake the tomatoes for 20 minutes. Remove the foil, pour the remaining wine over the tomatoes, and continue baking for 10 minutes. Let cool for 5 minutes and serve with the wine drippings over the top. |

*Per serving:* Calories 236 (From Fat 36); Fat 4g (Saturated 2g); Cholesterol 8mg; Sodium 197mg; Carbohydrate 34g (Dietary Fiber 2g); Protein 8g.

# Golden Pilaf

**Prep time:** 10 min • **Cook time:** 25 min • **Yield:** 6 servings

| Ingredients | Directions |
|---|---|
| **2 teaspoons olive oil**<br>**1 medium onion, chopped**<br>**¼ cup golden raisins** | *1* In a 2-quart saucepan, heat the olive oil over medium-high heat. Add the onions and raisins and sauté for 3 minutes. |
| **1 cup long-grain rice**<br>**½ teaspoon turmeric**<br>**⅛ teaspoon cinnamon**<br>**⅛ teaspoon cardamom** | *2* Stir in the rice, turmeric, cinnamon, and cardamom and sauté for 1 minute. Add the stock, bring the mixture to a boil, and cover. |
| **2 cups low-sodium chicken or vegetable stock**<br>**¼ cup pistachios, chopped**<br>**¼ cup parsley, chopped** | *3* Reduce the heat to a simmer for 15 to 18 minutes or until the liquid is fully absorbed. Meanwhile, toast the pistachios in a small nonstick skillet for 1 minute or until fragrant. Add the pistachios and parsley to the cooked rice and serve. |

***Per serving:*** *Calories 205 (From Fat 43); Fat 5g (Saturated 1g); Cholesterol 0mg; Sodium 48mg; Carbohydrate 36g (Dietary Fiber 2g); Protein 6g.*

# Bulgur Salad with White Beans and Spinach

**Prep time:** 20 min, plus 30 min chilling time • **Cook time:** 5 min •
**Yield:** 8 servings

| Ingredients | Directions |
|---|---|
| ¾ cup bulgur<br><br>2 cups water<br><br>1 pound baby spinach, chopped<br><br>¼ cup fresh parsley, chopped<br><br>¼ cup fresh mint, chopped<br><br>¼ cup sundried tomatoes (packed in oil), finely chopped<br><br>One 14.5-ounce can cannellini beans, drained and rinsed<br><br>Zest and juice of 2 lemons<br><br>¼ cup olive oil<br><br>½ teaspoon ground cumin<br><br>¼ teaspoon coriander<br><br>1 clove garlic, crushed<br><br>½ teaspoon sea salt<br><br>½ teaspoon pepper | *1* In a 2-quart saucepan, boil the water. Pour in the bulgur, cover, and remove from the heat. Allow the bulgur to sit for 20 minutes.<br><br>*2* Meanwhile, toss together the spinach, parsley, mint, sun-dried tomatoes, and beans. In a small bowl, whisk the lemon juice and zest, olive oil, cumin, coriander, garlic, salt, and pepper.<br><br>*3* Add the spinach mixture to the bulgur and toss with a fork. Whisk the dressing and pour over the top of the bulgur/spinach mixture, stirring to mix. Cover and chill for 30 minutes to 1 hour prior to serving. |

*Per serving:* Calories 174 (From Fat 71); Fat 8g (Saturated 1g); Cholesterol 0mg;
Sodium 394mg; Carbohydrate 22g (Dietary Fiber 6g); Protein 7g.

# Spinach and Lentils with Feta

**Prep time:** 5 min • **Cook time:** 45 min • **Yield:** 6 servings

| Ingredients | Directions |
|---|---|
| ½ cup brown lentils<br><br>2 cups low-sodium vegetable stock<br><br>2 tablespoons olive oil<br><br>½ a medium onion, sliced<br><br>16 ounces frozen spinach, defrosted<br><br>2 cloves garlic, chopped<br><br>1 teaspoon curry powder<br><br>¼ teaspoon paprika<br><br>¼ cup feta, crumbled | *1* In a 2-quart stockpot, bring the stock and lentils to a boil over medium-high heat. Reduce the heat to a simmer and cook for 30 minutes or until tender.<br><br>*2* In a medium skillet, heat the olive oil over medium-high heat for 1 minute; add the onions and sauté for 5 minutes.<br><br>*3* Meanwhile, drain and squeeze the spinach dry over a colander. Add the spinach to the onions and continue sautéing for 3 minutes. Add the cooked lentils, garlic, curry, and paprika and cook for 5 minutes. Serve with crumbled feta over top. |

*Per serving:* Calories 153 (From Fat 59); Fat 7g (Saturated 2g); Cholesterol 6mg; Sodium 238mg; Carbohydrate 16g (Dietary Fiber 4g); Protein 8g.

*Vary It!* For a spicier version, add ¼ teaspoon of cayenne pepper when you add the spices.

# Beet and Kidney Bean Salad

**Prep time:** 12 min • **Cook time:** 15 min • **Yield:** 4 servings

| Ingredients | Directions |
|---|---|
| 4 beets, scrubbed and stems removed | *1* Fill a 2-quart stockpot with water and add the beets. Bring the water to a boil and reduce the heat to a simmer until the beets are fork tender (about 10 minutes). Strain in a colander and immediately put the beets in ice water to halt cooking. |
| One 14.5-ounce can kidney beans, drained and rinsed | |
| 4 green onions, chopped | |
| Juice of 1 lemon | *2* Allow the beets to chill for 3 minutes. Remove the skins of the beets (they should peel easily without the need for a paring knife). Cut the beets into thin half-moon shapes and set aside. |
| 2 tablespoons olive oil | |
| 1 tablespoon pomegranate syrup or juice | |
| Salt and pepper to taste | *3* In a serving dish, toss together the kidney beans, green onions, lemon juice, olive oil, and pomegranate syrup and toss gently to mix. Add the beets, season with salt and pepper to taste, and serve. |

*Per serving:* Calories 175 (From Fat 67); Fat 7g (Saturated 1g); Cholesterol 0mg; Sodium 200mg; Carbohydrate 22g (Dietary Fiber 7g); Protein 6g.

*Note:* You can serve this bean salad at room temperature or chilled.

# Savory Fava Beans with Warm Pita Bread

**Prep time:** 10 min • **Cook time:** 15 min • **Yield:** 4 servings

| Ingredients | Directions |
|---|---|
| 1½ tablespoons olive oil | *1* In a large nonstick skillet, heat the olive oil over medium-high heat for 30 seconds. Add the onion, tomato, and garlic and sauté for 3 minutes, until soft. Add the fava beans and their liquid and bring to a boil. |
| 1 large onion, chopped | |
| 1 large tomato, diced | |
| 1 clove garlic, crushed | |
| One 15-ounce can fava beans, undrained | *2* Reduce the heat to medium and add the cumin, parsley, and lemon juice and season with the salt, pepper, and ground red pepper to taste. Cook for 5 minutes on medium heat. |
| 1 teaspoon ground cumin | |
| ¼ cup chopped fresh parsley | |
| ¼ cup lemon juice | *3* Meanwhile, heat the pita in a cast-iron skillet over medium-low heat until warm (1 to 2 minutes per side). Serve the warm pita with the fava beans (either on the side or loaded up with the bean mixture). |
| Salt and pepper to taste | |
| Crushed red pepper flakes, to taste | |
| 4 whole-grain pita bread pockets | |

*Per serving: Calories 325 (From Fat 64); Fat 7g (Saturated 1g); Cholesterol 0mg; Sodium 831mg; Carbohydrate 56g (Dietary Fiber 10g); Protein 13g.*

# Falafel

**Prep time:** 12 min • **Cook time:** 35 min • **Yield:** 6 servings

| Ingredients | Directions |
|---|---|
| **Two 14.5-ounce cans chickpeas, drained and rinsed** | *1* In a food processor, pulse the chickpeas, onion, parsley, cilantro, salt, red pepper flakes, garlic, and cumin for 3 minutes, stopping every 30 seconds to stir the mixture for even mixing. |
| **½ a large onion, roughly chopped (about 1 cup)** | |
| **2 tablespoons finely chopped fresh parsley** | *2* Combine the baking powder and flour in a small bowl. Remove the chickpea mixture from the food processor, stir in the flour mixture, and form the bean dough into twelve 3-inch patties. |
| **2 tablespoons finely chopped fresh cilantro** | |
| **½ teaspoon salt** | *3* Heat the oil in a skillet over medium-high heat for 1 minute or until hot. Add the patties, being careful not to crowd the pan. Pan-fry the patties for 3 to 4 minutes on each side or until a golden crust is formed. |
| **½ to 1 teaspoon red pepper flakes** | |
| **4 cloves garlic, minced** | |
| **1 teaspoon ground cumin** | *4* Serve hot or at room temperature. Serve with 1 to 2 tablespoons of Cucumber Yogurt Sauce. |
| **1 teaspoon baking powder** | |
| **¼ cup flour** | |
| **2 tablespoons olive oil** | |
| **Cucumber Yogurt Sauce for serving (see recipe earlier in this chapter)** | |

*Per serving:* Calories 207 (From Fat 62); Fat 7g (Saturated 1g); Cholesterol 0mg; Sodium 465mg; Carbohydrate 29g (Dietary Fiber 7g); Protein 8g.

# Chapter 7

# Starting and Ending with Style: Appetizers and Desserts

. . . . . . . . . . . . . . . . . . . .

### In This Chapter

▶ Creating big flavors in small dishes

▶ Satisfying your sweet tooth

. . . . . . . . . . . . . . . . . . . .

*T*apas, *meze,* and *antipasti* are all terms for small dishes served in the Mediterranean; we call them *appetizers*. Such small dishes are often served as a snack between work and dinnertime, and some people serve several appetizers at once as the dinner meal.

For after-dinner treats, people in the Mediterranean indulge in items that tend to be healthier than the processed desserts that are staples in other parts of the world. The dessert menu often includes an abundance of nuts, apricots, dates, lemons, and oranges.

This chapter shows you simple Mediterranean-style appetizers you can use as snacks or for your next party. It also presents some delicious dessert recipes that incorporate ingredients you can feel good about.

# *Toasted Almonds*

**Prep time:** 4 min • **Cook time:** 30 min • **Yield:** 16 servings

| *Ingredients* | *Directions* |
|---|---|
| **4 cups whole, raw almonds**<br><br>**1 egg white**<br><br>**1 tablespoon water**<br><br>**¼ teaspoon cayenne pepper**<br><br>**¼ teaspoon ground cumin**<br><br>**½ tablespoon sea salt** | *1* Preheat the oven to 300 degrees. Place the almonds in a medium bowl and set aside. In a small bowl, whisk the egg white and water until the egg is broken up. Pour the egg mixture over the almonds and stir. Add the spices and salt and stir until well blended. |
| | *2* Place the almonds on a baking sheet and bake, stirring every 10 minutes, for 30 to 40 minutes or until just toasted and you begin to smell the toasted nuts. Don't let the almonds get too dark, or they'll taste burnt. |
| | *3* Remove almonds from the oven and immediately transfer them to a heat-proof plate; allow the nuts to cool in a single layer. Serve at room temperature. |

*Per serving:* Calories 205 (From Fat 158); Fat 18g (Saturated 1g); Cholesterol 0mg; Sodium 222mg; Carbohydrate 8g (Dietary Fiber 4g); Protein 8g.

*Note:* Store in a glass container in the refrigerator and use within 1 to 2 weeks for best quality.

# *Toasted Pita Chips*

**Prep time:** 5 min • **Cook time:** 12–15 min • **Yield:** 4 servings

| Ingredients | Directions |
|---|---|
| **4 whole wheat pitas**<br>**4 teaspoons olive oil**<br>**Sea salt to taste** | *1* Preheat the oven to 375 degrees. |
| | *2* Using a pastry brush, brush each pita with 1 teaspoon of olive oil. Sprinkle with sea salt to taste. |
| | *3* Cut each pita into 8 wedges. Arrange the pita wedges on a baking sheet and bake for 12 to 15 minutes. Cool the pita chips to room temperature and serve. |

**Per serving:** *Calories 210 (From Fat 55); Fat 6g (Saturated 1g); Cholesterol 0mg; Sodium 341mg; Carbohydrate 35g (Dietary Fiber 5g); Protein 6g.*

**Note:** Serve with Hummus, Baba Gannoujh, or the healthy dip of your choice.

# *Hummus*

**Prep time:** 10 min • **Yield:** 16 servings

| *Ingredients* | *Directions* |
| --- | --- |
| **Two 14.5-ounce cans chickpeas** <br><br> **Juice of 2 lemons** <br><br> **2 cloves garlic** | *1* Drain the chickpeas and reserve ¼ to ½ cup of the liquid. Place the chickpeas in a food processor and puree until smooth. |
| **¼ tablespoon olive oil** <br><br> **¼ cup tahini paste** <br><br> **½ teaspoon salt** <br><br> **Pinch of cayenne pepper** | *2* Add the remaining ingredients and blend until the mixture is creamy. If necessary, add the liquid reserved from the canned chickpeas to create desired creaminess. Transfer the hummus to a bowl and serve. |

*Per serving:* Calories 85 (From Fat 25); Fat 3g (Saturated 0g); Cholesterol 0mg; Sodium 228mg; Carbohydrate 12g (Dietary Fiber 2g); Protein 3g.

*Tip:* Serve with Toasted Pita Chips or fresh vegetables such as carrots.

*Note:* Tahini paste is paste made from ground sesame seeds. It is a major component in Hummus and other Middle Eastern dishes. You can find tahini paste at most grocery stores or specialty stores near the cooking oils or possibly in the ethnic sections of the store.

*Note:* Store hummus in a glass container in the refrigerator for up to a week. Cover the surface with a thin layer of olive oil before refrigerating.

# Roasted Eggplant Dip (Baba Gannoujh)

**Prep time:** 5 min • **Cook time:** 30 min • **Yield:** 16 servings

| *Ingredients* | *Directions* |
|---|---|
| **2 large eggplants** <br> **½ cup tahini paste** | *1* Preheat the oven to 450 degrees. Line a baking sheet with foil. |
| **2 cloves garlic** <br> **Juice of 2 lemons** <br> **3 tablespoons water** <br> **1 tablespoon extra-virgin olive oil** <br> **1 teaspoon salt** | *2* Poke the eggplant once with a fork on all sides to allow the steam to escape during cooking. Bake the eggplant on a baking sheet for about 30 minutes or until soft. Remove the eggplant from the oven and cool until you can comfortably touch it. |
| **2 tablespoons fresh parsley, chopped, for serving** | *3* Cut the eggplant in half. Scoop out the inside of the eggplant with a spoon, discarding the skin. |
|  | *4* Pulse the cooked eggplant in a food processor for 1 minute. Add the tahini, garlic, lemon juice, water, olive oil, and salt to the eggplant mixture and blend until you achieve a thicker consistency. Transfer to a serving bowl, garnish with the chopped parsley, and serve with pita chips. |

*Per serving: Calories 68 (From Fat 45); Fat 5g (Saturated 1g); Cholesterol 0mg; Sodium 149mg; Carbohydrate 6g (Dietary Fiber 3g); Protein 2g.*

# Goat Cheese with Honey and Fruit

**Prep time:** 12 min • **Yield:** 8 servings

| Ingredients | Directions |
|---|---|
| 32 whole-grain crackers | *1* Arrange the crackers on a serving dish. Spread each cracker with 1 tablespoon of goat cheese and top with an apricot, a fig, or a pear slice. |
| 8 ounces goat cheese | |
| 8 dried apricots | |
| 8 dried figs | |
| 1 pear, thinly sliced | *2* In a microwave safe bowl, heat the honey for 30 seconds; drizzle the honey over the fruit and crackers and serve. |
| 3 tablespoons honey | |

*Per serving: Calories 249 (From Fat 99); Fat 11g (Saturated 6g); Cholesterol 22mg; Carbohydrate 31g (Dietary Fiber 4g); Protein 9g.*

# *Tomato and Mozzarella Bites*

**Prep time:** 10 min • **Cook time:** 5 min • **Yield:** 16 servings

| Ingredients | Directions |
|---|---|
| ¾ **cup balsamic vinegar** | *1* In a small saucepan, cook the vinegar and pomegranate juice over medium heat until it reduces by half, approximately 5 minutes. |
| ¼ **cup pomegranate juice** | |
| **4 vine-ripened tomatoes, sliced ¼-inch thick** | *2* Meanwhile, layer the sliced tomatoes on a serving platter and sprinkle each with sea salt. Layer a basil leaf over each tomato and top with a mozzarella slice. Drizzle the olive oil and the balsamic pomegranate reduction over the tomato and mozzarella bites. |
| **Sea salt to taste** | |
| **16 fresh basil leaves** | |
| **1 pound fresh mozzarella cheese, sliced ¼-inch-thick** | |
| ¼ **cup olive oil** | *3* Pierce each mozzarella bite with a toothpick and serve. |

***Per serving:*** *Calories 133 (From Fat 88); Fat 10g (Saturated 4g); Cholesterol 22mg; Sodium 182mg; Carbohydrate 4g (Dietary Fiber 0g); Protein 7g.*

# *Italian Bruschetta*

**Prep time:** 12 min • **Cook Time:** 3 min • **Yield:** 16 servings

| *Ingredients* | *Directions* |
|---|---|
| **1 French baguette**<br>**¼ cup basil, chopped**<br>**6 Roma tomatoes, chopped**<br>**3 cloves garlic, chopped, plus 1 whole clove for rubbing**<br>**¼ cup olive oil**<br>**½ teaspoon salt** | *1* Cut the baguette into ½-inch-thick slices and place 6 inches under the broiler for 2 to 3 minutes until toasted. Watch the baguette so it doesn't burn. Once toasted, take out of the oven and set aside. |
| | *2* Combine the basil, tomatoes, chopped garlic, olive oil, and salt. |
| | *3* Cut the ends off the whole garlic clove. After the bread is done broiling, rub each piece with the garlic. Evenly spread the topping mixture on each slice of bread. |
| | *4* Arrange the slices on a platter or individual plates and serve immediately. |

*Per serving:* Calories 119 (From Fat 36); Fat 4g (Saturated 1g); Cholesterol 0mg; Sodium 265mg; Carbohydrate 17g (Dietary Fiber 1g); Protein 4g.

# *Pan-Grilled Shrimp*

**Prep time:** 15 min • **Cook time:** 8 min • **Yield:** 6 servings

| Ingredients | Directions |
|---|---|
| **24 raw shrimp, peeled and deveined (tail may be intact)** | *1* Skewer 4 shrimp ½ inch apart on each of 6 small skewers. |
| **8 cloves garlic, sliced** **¼ cup olive oil** **¼ teaspoon cracked red pepper flakes** **1 lemon, zested and cut into 6 wedges** | *2* Mix the garlic, olive oil, and cracked pepper in a small skillet. Heat the mixture over medium heat to infuse flavors, about 3 minutes. Remove from the heat and add the lemon zest. |
| **1 cup parsley, chopped** | *3* Using a pastry brush, brush both sides of the shrimp skewers with the heated oil mixture. |
| **Sea salt to taste** **Cracked black pepper to taste** | *4* Heat a grill pan, cast-iron pan, or griddle over medium-high heat. Cook the skewers 1-inch apart for 3 to 4 minutes on each side, or until pink in color. Sprinkle the shrimp evenly with parsley, sea salt, and cracked pepper and serve each with a lemon wedge. |

*Per serving:* Calories 111 (From Fat 85); Fat 9g (Saturated 1g); Cholesterol 36mg; Sodium 36mg; Carbohydrate 2g (Dietary Fiber 0g); Protein 5g.

# Ricotta Cake

**Prep time:** 35 min • **Cook time:** 45 min, plus cooling time • **Yield:** 12 servings

| Ingredients | Directions |
|---|---|
| 1 tablespoon plus ½ cup butter | *1* Preheat the oven to 325 degrees. Coat a springform cake pan with 1 tablespoon butter and dust evenly with 1 table-spoon of the flour. |
| 1 tablespoon plus ⅔ cup flour | |
| ¼ cup olive oil | *2* In a mixing bowl, beat the remaining butter, the olive oil, and the sugar until smooth and fluffy. In a separate mixing bowl, combine the remaining flour, the baking powder, and the salt and set aside. |
| ¾ cup sugar | |
| 2 teaspoons baking powder | |
| ⅛ teaspoon salt | |
| 4 eggs, separated | *3* In a third mixing bowl, beat the egg whites until stiff peaks form. Add the egg yolks, ricotta, and orange zest to the butter mixture and stir. Mix in the flour mixture until a smooth batter forms. |
| 1 cup lowfat ricotta cheese | |
| 3 tablespoons orange zest | |
| ¼ cup apricot preserves or jam | *4* Fold the egg whites into the cake batter and pour it into prepared pan. Bake the cake for 45 minutes or until done in the center. |
| ½ cup walnuts, chopped | |
| | *5* Cool for 25 minutes. Use a knife to sepa-rate the cake from the edges and then release the spring form. |
| | *6* In a small saucepan or microwave-safe dish, heat the apricot preserves until liquefied; add the walnuts and drizzle over the cake before serving. |

*Per serving:* Calories 266 (From Fat 158); Fat 18g (Saturated 7g); Cholesterol 29mg; Sodium 192mg; Carbohydrate 24g (Dietary Fiber 0g); Protein 5g.

# *Rice Pudding*

**Prep time:** 15 min • **Cook time:** 45 min • **Yield:** 6 servings

| Ingredients | Directions |
|---|---|
| ½ cup basmati rice | **1** Soak the rice in water for 10 minutes and drain. |
| 4 cups milk | |
| 3 tablespoons sugar | **2** In a heavy saucepan, bring the milk and sugar to a low boil over medium-high heat. Add the rice, raisins, cardamom, and cinnamon and simmer over low heat until thickened (about 45 minutes), stirring frequently. |
| ¼ cup raisins | |
| ½ teaspoon cardamom | |
| ¼ teaspoon cinnamon | |
| ½ teaspoon rose water (optional) | **3** Remove from the heat and add the rose water (if desired). Combine the almonds and orange zest. Ladle the pudding into serving bowls and garnish with the almond mixture. Serve hot or cold. |
| ¼ almonds, chopped | |
| 1 tablespoon orange zest | |

***Per serving:*** *Calories 207 (From Fat 43); Fat 5g (Saturated 1g); Cholesterol 8mg; Sodium 75mg; Carbohydrate 34g (Dietary Fiber 1g); Protein 8g.*

# Baked Farina

**Prep time:** 25 min • **Cook time:** 1 hr, plus cooling time • **Yield:** 24 servings

| Ingredients | Directions |
|---|---|
| **Nonstick cooking spray**<br>**8 cups milk**<br>**¼ cup butter**<br>**1 cup sugar**<br>**2 eggs**<br>**1¼ cup farina**<br>**1 teaspoon orange blossom water or vanilla extract**<br>**¼ cup honey**<br>**1 tablespoon water** | *1* Preheat the oven to 350 degrees. Spray a 9-x-13-inch pan with nonstick cooking spray. |
| | *2* In a large saucepan, heat the milk, butter, and sugar over medium-high heat until almost boiling. Stir frequently to avoid scalding or burning the milk. Meanwhile, in a medium mixing bowl, beat the eggs until fluffy. |
| | *3* Remove the milk mixture from the heat and add the farina, whisking constantly for 1 minute. Add the orange blossom water. Temper the eggs by slowly drizzling 1 cup of the hot milk mixture while beating. |
| | *4* Add the tempered egg mixture back into the milk mixture and whisk to blend. Pour the batter into the prepared pan and bake for 1 hour or until set and slightly golden on top. |
| | *5* In a microwave-safe bowl, heat the honey and water for 30 seconds or until thin and liquefied. Poke holes in the surface of the cake and drizzle the honey mixture over the surface. Cool the cake for 30 minutes before cutting and serving. |

***Per serving:*** *Calories 129 (From Fat 25); Fat 3g (Saturated 2g); Cholesterol 9mg; Sodium 54mg; Carbohydrate 22g (Dietary Fiber 0g); Protein 4g.*

***Note:*** Farina is a cereal grain made from wheat. You may know it better by its brand names, Cream of Wheat or Malt-o-Meal.

# *Panna Cotta*

**Prep time:** 15 min, plus chilling time • **Cook time:** 7 min • **Yield:** 4 servings

| *Ingredients* | *Directions* |
|---|---|
| **1 teaspoon unflavored gelatin**<br><br>**¾ cup plus 2 tablespoons heavy whipping cream**<br><br>**3 tablespoons whole milk**<br><br>**2 tablespoons sugar**<br><br>**2 tablespoons honey**<br><br>**1 cup blackberries, strawberries, or raspberries** | *1* In a small bowl, sprinkle the gelatin over ¼ cup of the cream. Allow the mixture to stand for 1 minute to soften the gelatin. |
| | *2* In a heavy saucepan, combine the remaining cream, milk, and sugar. Bring the mixture to a boil over medium heat while continuously stirring. Remove the mixture from the heat and whisk in the gelatin mixture until the gelatin dissolves. |
| | *3* Pour the mixture into 4 small custard cups and chill for at least 4 hours. |
| | *4* To serve, unmold the panna cotta onto serving plates. Drizzle honey over each panna cotta and serve with the berries. |

*Per serving: Calories 260 (From Fat 179); Fat 20g (Saturated 12g); Cholesterol 73mg; Sodium 32mg; Carbohydrate 21g (Dietary Fiber 2g); Protein 2g.*

# Crepes with Berries

**Prep time:** 5 min, plus chilling time • **Cook time:** 12 min • **Yield:** 8 servings

| Ingredients | Directions |
|---|---|
| 2 eggs | **1** Combine the eggs, milk, flour, salt, and butter in a blender until smooth, about 2 minutes. Cover and refrigerate the batter for 1 hour. |
| 1 cup milk | |
| ⅔ cup flour | |
| ⅛ teaspoon salt | |
| 1 tablespoon butter, melted | **2** In a small bowl, gently combine the berries and sugar. Cover and set aside at room temperature. Spray a nonstick skillet with nonstick cooking spray and heat over medium heat. |
| 1½ cups strawberries, blackberries, raspberries, and/or blueberries | |
| 2 tablespoons sugar | **3** Ladle ¼ cup of the batter into the skillet and quickly rotate and coat the pan with the batter to make a thin crepe. |
| Nonstick cooking spray | |
| Powdered sugar for dusting | **4** Cook for 1 minute (look for golden brown edges) and then flip and cook for 30 seconds or until golden. Remove from the pan, place on a plate, and cover with a warm towel. |
| | **5** Repeat Steps 3 and 4 with the remaining batter. Fold each crepe in half and then in half again. Top each crepe with berries and dust with powdered sugar to serve. |

*Per serving:* Calories 108 (From Fat 17); Fat 2g (Saturated 1g); Cholesterol 5mg; Sodium 73mg; Carbohydrate 19g (Dietary Fiber 1g); Protein 3g.

# *Lemon Ices*

**Prep time:** 5 min, plus freezing time 2 hours • **Yield:** 6 servings

| Ingredients | Directions |
|---|---|
| **2 cups water** <br> **¾ cup sugar** <br> **Zest and juice of 5 lemons** | **1** Heat the sugar and water in a heavy saucepan over medium heat until the sugar has dissolved. Add the lemon zest and juice and stir to combine. |
| | **2** Pour the mixture into a 9-x-13-inch glass baking dish. Freeze the mixture until all the liquid is gone, scraping every 20 minutes. During the last hour of freezing, scrape every 10 minutes to create a finer ice. Spoon into cups and serve. |

*Per serving:* Calories 107 (From Fat 0); Fat 0g (Saturated 0g); Cholesterol 0mg; Sodium 1mg; Carbohydrate 28g (Dietary Fiber 0g); Protein 0g.

*Tip:* For a smoother consistency, you can chill the lemon mixture in an ice-cream maker. Both methods are considered traditional depending on the area of the Mediterranean.

# Orange Cardamom Cookies

**Prep time:** 15 min, plus chilling time • **Cook time:** 30 min • **Yield:** 48 servings

| Ingredients | Directions |
|---|---|
| **3 cups flour** <br> **¾ teaspoon baking soda** <br> **1 teaspoon cream of tartar** <br> **½ teaspoon plus 1 teaspoon cardamom** <br> **½ teaspoon salt** | *1* In a large mixing bowl, whisk together the flour, baking soda, cream of tartar, ½ teaspoon of the cardamom, and the salt. Set aside. |
| **1 stick room-temperature butter** <br> **1½ cups plus ¾ cup sugar** <br> **2 eggs** <br> **½ teaspoon orange blossom water or vanilla extract** | *2* Using a stand mixer, cream the butter and 1½ cups of the sugar until creamy, about 4 minutes. Add the eggs and mix for 1 minute. Add the orange blossom water, orange zest, and milk and gently mix for 1 minute. |
| **1 tablespoon orange zest** <br> **¼ cup milk** | *3* Mix the flour mixture into the batter just until combined. Chill the dough in the refrigerator for at least 1 hour. |
| | *4* Combine the remaining sugar and cardamom. Roll the chilled dough into 1-inch balls. Roll the dough in the cardamom sugar and place each ball about 2 inches apart on a baking sheet. |
| | *5* Bake the cookies for 10 to 12 minutes or until the edges are slightly golden brown. Allow the cookies to cool on the baking sheet for 3 minutes and then transfer to a cooling rack. Serve. |

***Per serving:*** *Calories 83 (From Fat 18); Fat 2g (Saturated 1g); Cholesterol 5mg; Sodium 61mg; Carbohydrate 15g (Dietary Fiber 0g); Protein 1g.*

# Chapter 8

# Ten Tips for Getting More Plant-Based Foods in Your Diet

. . . . . . . . . . . . . . . . . . . . . . . . . . . . . . .

### In This Chapter

▶ Upping your intake of fruits, veggies, and herbs

▶ Eating whole grains and legumes every day

. . . . . . . . . . . . . . . . . . . . . . . . . . . . . . .

*T*he biggest concept behind a Mediterranean-style diet is adding more plant-based foods, such as fruits, vegetables, herbs, legumes, and even whole grains, to every meal. Fruits and vegetables are the main components of this push; you want to have five to nine servings of fruits and vegetables each day. Hitting that number may be a simple change for some people, but it may be a bigger challenge for others. Similarly, you may be at a loss as to how legumes, herbs, and whole grains can fit into your lifestyle.

When you aren't used to eating many fruits, vegetables, and the like, knowing how to add them to your diet may be quite difficult. Fortunately, adding plant-based foods to your diet isn't rocket science. This chapter is here to help make the shift effortless and tasty.

Increasing the variety of the plant-based foods you eat each day means you also get a good variety of the nutrients your body needs.

# Keeping Sliced Vegetables on Hand

One of the easiest ways to consume more veggies is to eat them raw as snacks. The key to making it simple is to pre-slice a bunch of different vegetables, such as bell peppers, broccoli, carrots, and any other favorites, for the week at one time. Then you can grab some of the veggies and your favorite healthy dip, such as hummus, while sitting at your desk or watching a movie for an instant snack.

In addition, you can throw whatever cut veggies you don't use as snacks into a soup, pasta dish, salad, or some scrambled eggs.

# Including a Fruit or Vegetable with Every Meal

Planning to have a fruit or vegetable with every meal is a good mindset to get you into the Mediterranean spirit. After you have this little mental guideline in your head, you can find all sorts of creative ways to make it happen. For example, you can spruce up your sandwich with dark leafy greens and tomatoes, add some fruit to your yogurt, or slice up some raw veggies to have on hand as a snack.

You can make this habit work for you in all kinds of ways. Chapter 5 introduces a sampling of recipes for main dishes for every meal, many of which are heavy on the veggies. Most of the delicious side dishes we present in Chapter 6 incorporate vegetables as well. And you even find fruits and veggies well-represented in the appetizers and desserts we suggest trying in Chapter 7.

By focusing on this guideline, you'll naturally start incorporating five to nine servings of fruits and vegetables during the day.

## *Keeping a Fruit Bowl on Your Counter*

Rather than the old mantra "out of sight, out of mind," you want to go for "in sight, in mind." Keep a fruit bowl on your counter to remind you to eat some fruit during the day with your meals or snacks. If you have kids, you may be surprised how much more fruit they eat when it's in plain sight. Having a bowl of fresh fruit also looks beautiful and sets the stage for your kitchen to be a healthy, nutritious spot.

Don't just settle for a few bananas; fill the bowl up with all kinds of fresh, seasonal fruit so that you have choices and aren't left with the same type of fruit all day.

## *Adding Fruit to Your Cereals*

Adding fruit to your cereals is a great strategy that gives your meal more flavor and makes it more satisfying. Slice up any sort of fresh fruit, such as bananas, nectarines, or peaches, or sprinkle some fresh berries on your cereal or oatmeal. Dried fruit is also a wonderful choice and is easy to store in your pantry. Just choose dried fruits with no added sugars.

You can add fresh fruit to your cereal year-round. Just keep frozen fruits and berries in your freezer so you can thaw them in the microwave in a few seconds. Their warm, juicy texture is perfect on top of oatmeal or low-fat granola.

## Dressing Up Your Salad with Fresh Fruits and Vegetables

Don't settle for a boring old leafy green salad. You can create a savory or sweet masterpiece by incorporating some fruits and veggies. For example, add sliced bell peppers, tomatoes, and fresh herbs, such as dill, for a savory experience. Sweeten up another salad by adding mandarin orange slices along with some walnuts.

Salads in general are a great way to up your plant food intake. Use salads frequently as an additional vegetable side or as your entree with some kind of protein (such as chicken or egg). For inspiration, see the recipes in Chapter 5 for the Char-Grilled Chicken with Feta over Mixed Greens and the Grilled Salmon with Carmelized Onions over Mixed Greens.

## Sneaking Veggies and Herbs into Your Egg Dishes

You can use vegetables to add tons of flavor and texture to the most basic egg dishes, such as scrambled eggs. Chop up fresh tomatoes (okay, those are technically a fruit), fresh spinach, onions, or even zucchini. If you have leftover steamed veggies, they're perfect to throw into an egg dish the next morning. You can also add fresh herbs to the mix to add significant flavor. Basil, parsley, and oregano are all great flavors with eggs. Fresh salsa is also an excellent addition to egg dishes.

For some recipe ideas, check out Chapter 5, where we walk you through making a Vegetable Omelet, Zucchini and Goat Cheese Frittata, and Dilled Eggs.

And remember that egg dishes don't just have to be for breakfast; they can be great, quick meal ideas for lunch and dinner, too.

# Punching Up Your Pasta with Fresh Produce

Pasta dishes are the perfect food to add fresh vegetables and herbs to. Even if you already use a vegetable-based sauce such as marinara, you can up the vegetable quotient by adding blanched broccoli, carrots, and bell peppers. Doing so adds more variety and helps you eat less pasta than you may otherwise.

And don't forget about herbs! Fresh herbs can turn your pasta dish into something spectacular. Experiment and see what types of blends work well for you. One idea: Next time you're eating a pasta salad, try adding some fresh basil leaves.

See our recipes for Puttanesca and Baked Eggplant Parmesan with Linguini in Chapter 5 for some pasta inspiration.

# Starting Off with a Little Vegetable Soup

Beginning a meal with a cup of healthy soup is an easy strategy for adding more vegetables and helping with weight management. Use low-calorie vegetable or tomato soup as a starter for your meals. The soup can help you feel full and satisfied so that you eat less of the main meal.

# Supercharging Soups and Stews with Whole Grains

You can add some flavor and texture to soups and stews by incorporating whole grains such as whole-wheat pasta or pearl barley into them. Adding whole grains to plain vegetable soup can recreate a side dish as a complete meal. Whole grains provide fiber and other healthful nutrients and add to the variety of plant-based foods you take in during your day.

# Adding Beans to, Well, Everything

Beans are versatile, flavorful, and easy to use with many different dishes. Look for ways to include them every day. For some great side dishes that focus on legumes, turn to Chapter 6.

 Always keep some dried and canned beans on hand in your pantry. You can rinse canned beans and add them to soups, stews, salads, pasta dishes, or grain dishes.

### Apple & Mac

iPad For Dummies,
5th Edition
978-1-118-49823-1

iPhone 5 For
Dummies, 6th Edition
978-1-118-35201-4

MacBook For
Dummies, 4th Edition
978-1-118-20920-2

OS X Mountain Lion
For Dummies
978-1-118-39418-2

### Blogging & Social Media

Facebook For
Dummies, 4th Edition
978-1-118-09562-1

Mom Blogging
For Dummies
978-1-118-03843-7

Pinterest
For Dummies
978-1-118-32800-2

WordPress For
Dummies, 5th Edition
978-1-118-38318-6

### Business

Commodities
For Dummies,
2nd Edition
978-1-118-01687-9

Investing For
Dummies, 6th Edition
978-0-470-90545-6

Personal Finance
For Dummies,
7th Edition
978-1-118-11785-9

QuickBooks 2013
For Dummies
978-1-118-35641-8

Small Business
Marketing Kit
For Dummies,
3rd Edition
978-1-118-31183-7

### Careers

Job Interviews For
Dummies, 4th Edition
978-1-118-11290-8

Job Searching with
Social Media
For Dummies
978-0-470-93072-4

Personal Branding
For Dummies
978-1-118-11792-7

Resumes For
Dummies, 6th Edition
978-0-470-87361-8

Success as a
Mediator
For Dummies
978-1-118-07862-4

### Diet & Nutrition

Belly Fat Diet
For Dummies
978-1-118-34585-6

Eating Clean
For Dummies
978-1-118-00013-7

Nutrition For
Dummies, 5th Edition
978-0-470-93231-5

### Digital Photography

Digital Photography
For Dummies,
7th Edition
978-1-118-09203-3

Digital SLR Cameras
& Photography For
Dummies, 4th Edition
978-1-118-14489-3

Photoshop Elements
11 For Dummies
978-1-118-40821-6

### Gardening

Herb Gardening
For Dummies,
2nd Edition
978-0-470-61778-6

Vegetable Gardening
For Dummies,
2nd Edition
978-0-470-49870-5

### Health

Anti-Inflammation
Diet For Dummies
978-1-118-02381-5

Diabetes
For Dummies,
3rd Edition
978-0-470-27086-8

Living Paleo
For Dummies
978-1-118-29405-5

### Hobbies

Beekeeping
For Dummies
978-0-470-43065-1

eBay For Dummies,
7th Edition
978-1-118-09806-6

Raising Chickens
For Dummies
978-0-470-46544-8

Wine For Dummies,
5th Edition
978-1-118-28872-6

Writing Young Adult
Fiction For Dummies
978-0-470-94954-2

### Language & Foreign Language

500 Spanish Verbs
For Dummies
978-1-118-02382-2

English Grammar
For Dummies,
2nd Edition
978-0-470-54664-2

French All-in One
For Dummies
978-1-118-22815-9

German Essentials
For Dummies
978-1-118-18422-6

Italian For Dummies,
2nd Edition
978-1-118-00465-4

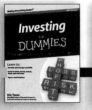
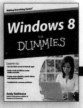

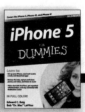

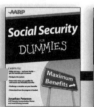
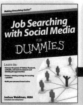
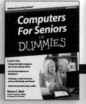
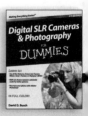

# Take Dummies with you everywhere you go!

Whether you're excited about e-books, want more from the web, must have your mobile apps, or swept up in social media, Dummies makes everything easier .

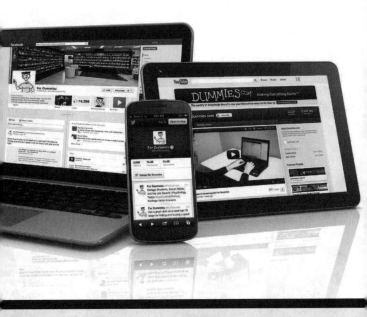

**Visit Us**

**Like Us**

**Follow Us**

**Watch Us**

**Join Us**

**Pin Us**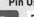

**Circle Us**

**Shop Us**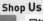

# Dummies products make life easier!

- DIY
- Consumer Electronics
- Crafts
- Software
- Cookware

- Hobbies
- Videos
- Music
- Games
- and More!

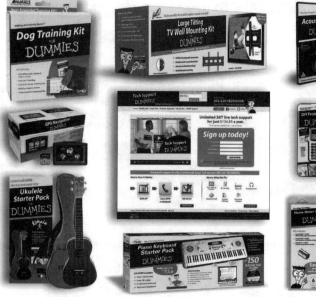

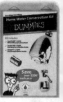

For more information, go to **Dummies.com®** and search the store by category.

FOR
DUMMIES
A Wiley Brand